Mastering Medicare Insurance for Starters:

RESEARCHED METHODS, RESOURCES, AND GUIDANCE

FOR NEW MEDICARE RECIPIENTS

AUTHOR: J.M RICHARDSON

Table Of Contents

MEDICARE ESSENTIALS

Professional Reference:

If you have any questions at all, do not hesitate to email or call Roxanne Robertson. She is a verified Medicare insurance consultant, licensed in over 40 states. Roxanne specializes in current Medicare options, and resources which has personally helped thousands of Medicare recipients just like you. In addition her service is free.

She can be reached at:

Roxanne@medigapselect.com

Or directly on her personal cell (913)-592-1291 text is also an option.

9:00 A.M - 6:00 P.M Monday-Saturday

What Is Medicare?

Simply put, Medicare is government-sponsored health care that came to pass as part of the Social Security Amendments of 1965. President Lyndon B. Johnson signed the program into law but his predecessor, President Harry S. Truman, was the true visionary behind the program. Not only was Truman called the "daddy of Medicare" but he also was the first person to enroll in the program.

Initially intended to provide care for those on Social Security, Medicare has evolved to become the main source of health coverage for people 65 years and older in this country. In the 1970s, the program expanded to include coverage for people with long-term disabilities, regardless of their age.

Medicare acts like private health insurance. From that endorsement alone, it should be easy to see that Medicare is not free. Like an insurance company, there are premiums and out-of-pocket expenses that you, the beneficiary, will be expected to pay.

Medicare Eligibility

To be eligible for Medicare, you must first be a U.S. citizen or have been a permanent legal resident of the country for at least five years. Specifically, permanent U.S. residents must hold a valid Green Card for at least five years and must live in the United States for the five years immediately preceding their application for Medicare.

Citizens and qualifying legal residents older than 65 years old are eligible for Medicare. Individuals with certain medical disabilities may also be eligible, regardless of their age.

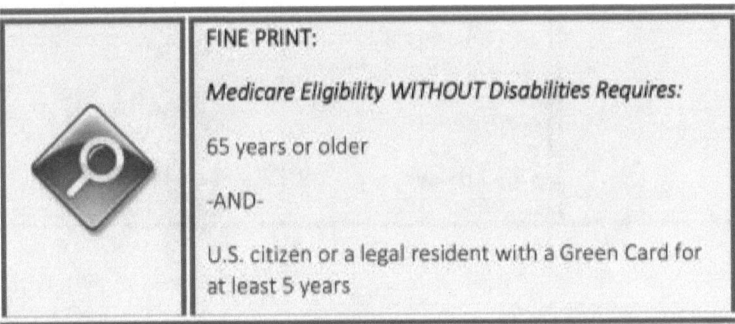

FINE PRINT:

Medicare Eligibility WITHOUT Disabilities Requires:

65 years or older

-AND-

U.S. citizen or a legal resident with a Green Card for at least 5 years

Medicare payroll taxes play a role in how much you will pay for Medicare coverage but do not determine your eligibility for the program, not unless kidney disease comes into play. Medicare-eligible employment simply means that you or your spouse paid Medicare taxes to the government over a defined period of time. This will be discussed further in Chapter 3.

An individual who has permanent kidney failure, also known as end-stage renal disease (ESRD), is eligible for Medicare at any age if he or she needs dialysis or is in need of or has had a kidney transplant, though that alone is not enough to get onto Medicare's roster.

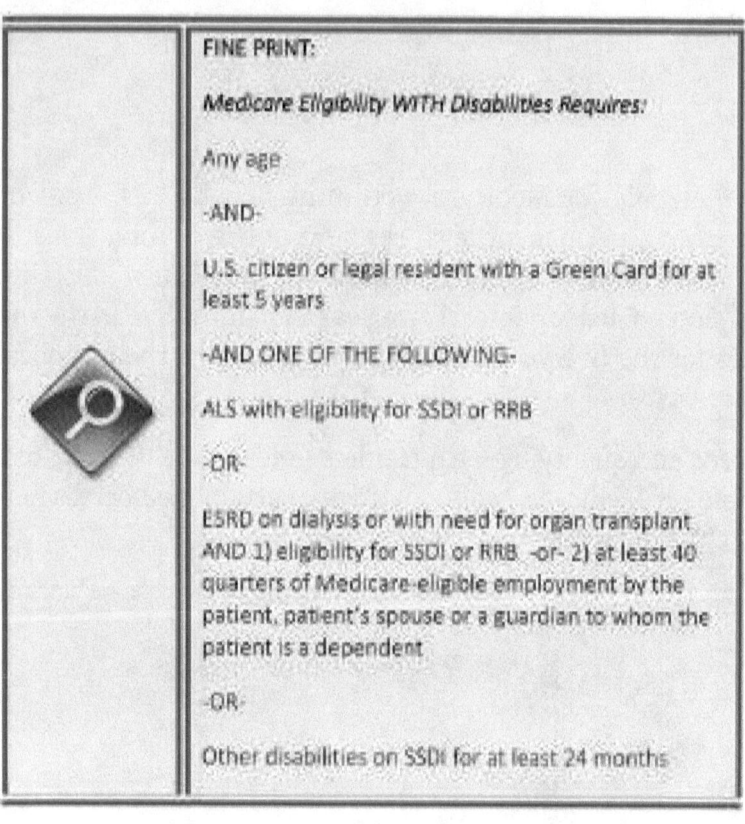

FINE PRINT:

Medicare Eligibility WITH Disabilities Requires:

Any age

-AND-

U.S. citizen or legal resident with a Green Card for at least 5 years

-AND ONE OF THE FOLLOWING-

ALS with eligibility for SSDI or RRB

-OR-

ESRD on dialysis or with need for organ transplant AND 1) eligibility for SSDI or RRB -or- 2) at least 40 quarters of Medicare-eligible employment by the patient, patient's spouse or a guardian to whom the patient is a dependent

-OR-

Other disabilities on SSDI for at least 24 months

Additional criteria must be met that includes one of the following:

- He or she has worked the required amount of time in a job that paid taxes to Medicare.

- He or she is eligible for or is receiving Social Security Disability Insurance (SSDI) or Railroad Retirement Board (RRB) benefits.

- He or she is the spouse or dependent child of someone who meets the criteria for #1 or #2.

Amyotrophic lateral sclerosis (ALS) is more commonly known as Lou Gehrig's disease. People with this condition are eligible for Medicare benefits once they also meet eligibility criteria for SSDI or RRB.

People with other disabilities do not meet eligibility criteria until they have been on SSDI for a minimum of 24 months. Medicare benefits may begin in the 25th month. Eligibility is taken away if their SSDI is discontinued for any reason.

If someone becomes eligible for SSDI a second time, they cannot sign back up for Medicare where they left off. They will have to wait another 24 months before they are eligible for Medicare coverage again.

The A, B, C, D of Medicare

Medicare services are divided across four categories – A, B, C and D. Medicare Parts A and B are often called "Original" Medicare, not only because they cover the "nuts and bolts" of your healthcare needs, but because they were the only parts of Medicare that existed back in 1965. Medicare Parts C and D came to pass in 1997 and 2003, respectively.

Medicare Part A covers hospital and emergency care. These services can extend beyond hospital walls to include rehabilitation facilities, nursing homes, hospice and home healthcare offerings. Nothing is ever black and white: certain criteria must be met in order for Medicare to pay for these services.

Medicare Part B covers outpatient care such as ambulance rides, counseling, diabetic supplies, doctor visits, imaging studies, laboratory tests, medical equipment, medications (a VERY limited number), physical therapy, preventive screening tests and vaccinations (in certain cases). Preventive services are intended to stop diseases from developing in the first place or to identify diseases in their earlier stages to allow for more effective treatment early on.

Medicare Part C is known as Medicare Advantage and can substitute for Original Medicare. These optional plans allow enrollees to purchase healthcare coverage from private insurance companies approved by Medicare. This may allow you to get extra healthcare coverage beyond what Parts A and B offer. Depending on the Medicare Advantage plan selected. Some of these plans may be more cost effective for certain individuals as they combine Part A, Part B and sometimes Part D coverage into one plan.

Medicare Part D covers outpatient prescription medications and, similarly to Part C, is offered through private insurance companies approved by Medicare. Each plan has different associated costs depending on how narrow or broad the drug coverage is. It is important to note that medications used during an inpatient hospital stay are covered under Part A. A limited number of medications are covered by Part B.

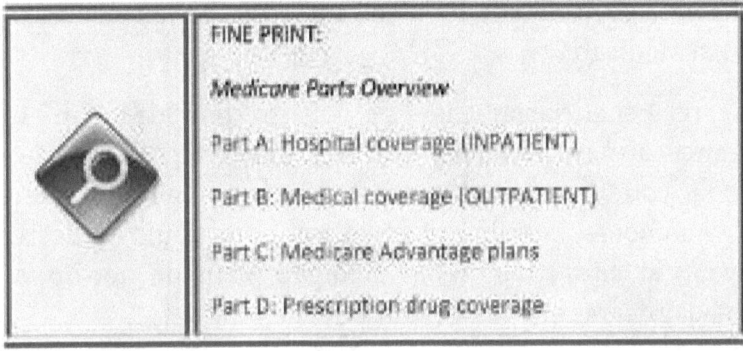

FINE PRINT:

Medicare Parts Overview

Part A: Hospital coverage (INPATIENT)

Part B: Medical coverage (OUTPATIENT)

Part C: Medicare Advantage plans

Part D: Prescription drug coverage

Medicare Supplement Plans, aka Medigap

Medigap plans may sound like they are an official part of Medicare, but they are not. They are optional Medicare Supplemental Insurance plans that have been standardized by the federal government to cover some of the left-over costs of Original Medicare.

Medicare beneficiaries may be left to pay deductibles, co-insurance, and co-payments for certain services. A Medigap plan can help you to save on those costs. Depending on the Medigap plan you choose, certain out of pocket costs could be decreased or even cut altogether. What Medigap plans do not do is add more healthcare services to your coverage.

Except for Massachusetts, Minnesota, and Wisconsin, states offer Medigap plans that are standardized according to a letter system (plans A-N). Plans with a particular letter offer the exact same coverage. The only difference between specific lettered plans will be cost. If you are interested in a Medigap plan, be sure to shop around for the best price but make sure you pick a company with good customer service.

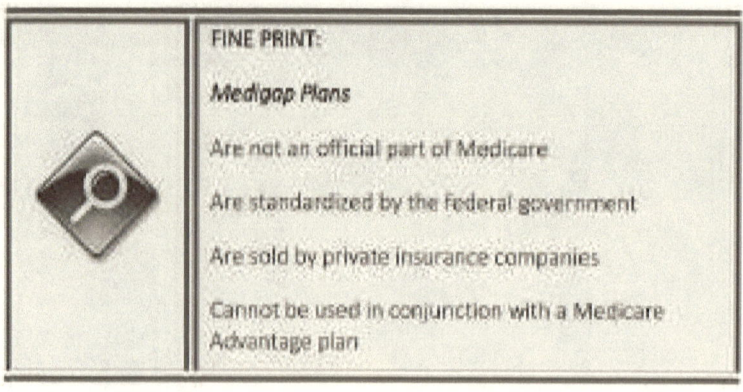

FINE PRINT:

Medigap Plans

Are not an official part of Medicare

Are standardized by the federal government

Are sold by private insurance companies

Cannot be used in conjunction with a Medicare Advantage plan

One of the most important things to know about Medigap plans is that you cannot have one if you also have a Medicare Advantage plan. This leaves you with an important choice. Which will be worth more to you in the long run – saving money on deductibles, co-insurance, and co-payments with a Medigap plan or adding additional services to your healthcare coverage with a Medicare Advantage plan?

The Affordable Care Act and Medicare

If there is one thing that has been said time and again by the Obama administration, it is that Medicare would not be affected by the Affordable Care Act (ACA) of 2010, commonly referred to as Obamacare. Since Medicare is not part of the Health Insurance Marketplace set forth by the ACA, eligibility for the program remains untouched. Coverage to Medicare beneficiaries has not been cut.

Despite the rhetoric, changes have indeed taken place since the ACA passed that have impacted Medicare.

Supporters of the ACA find that Medicare has actually been strengthened by the health law.

Improving hospital care: Medicare is not only about what care you receive but about the quality of that care. Obamacare has put legislation in place that penalizes hospitals that do not meet certain quality measures. Hospital readmissions fall under this category. If you are readmitted to the hospital within a short period of time for the same or a related medical problem, it implies the hospital may not have done enough to stabilize you before they discharged you. The ACA fines hospitals for frequent short-term readmissions, incentivizing those hospitals to improve quality of care.

Prescription drug coverage: Medicare Part D has a coverage gap, the infamous "donut hole". It is called a hole because your plan coverage drops off after you have spent a certain amount of money on prescription medications in a given year. Obamacare aims to close this coverage gap by 2020. It also has negotiated with pharmaceutical companies so that you get 50 percent discounts on all brand name medications when you are in the donut hole. Are you confused by the donut hole? These and other issues will be addressed in Chapter 4.

Preventive screening services: Medicare coverage has expanded to include preventive services such as Wellness Visits and screening tests such as mammograms and colonoscopies—for free! After all, an ounce of prevention is worth a pound of cure. It all comes down to medical necessity. These magic words have become the focus for all of healthcare. Understanding how to make the most out of these services will be the focus of Chapter 5.

Targeting Medicare fraud: Uncovering Medicare fraud could save billions of dollars for the Medicare Trust Fund, preserving Medicare for years to come. The ACA created the Health Care Fraud and Abuse Control Program which recovered more than $10.7 billion in its first 3 years alone. Before 2010, Medicare funds were expected to last through 2017; the ACA to date has extended this to at least 2028.

That does not mean that all things have been positive.

Paying for Hospital Stays: Medicare still covers your hospital stay but has changed how it pays for it in some cases. The end result could mean savings for Medicare but a bigger bill for you. Learn about the 2-Midnight Rule in Chapter 7.

Medicare Funding: Obamacare took $716 billion away from Medicare to put its plan into action. The Obama administration claims those funds were re-directed back into Medicare to make it more efficient and solvent. Has it worked?

Controversy has surrounded Obamacare since its inception in 2010. Regardless of your political affiliation, understanding how the law has impacted Medicare will help you to understand how the program works today.

MEDICARE COSTS

Medicare Taxes

Most people have paid well in advance for Medicare. Dollars are taken paycheck after paycheck with the promise that Medicare will provide coverage to you once you reach eligibility age. How long, rather than how much, you pay into the system decides how much you will have to pay out of pocket when the time comes to use the program.

The Medicare Tax is applied to your earned income, minus any pre-tax deductions. It does not apply to capital gains and other investment income. In 1966, the Medicare Tax began at a modest rate of 0.7 percent. Today, the payroll tax is increased to 2.9 percent.

How much you pay in taxes depends on your employment status. People who are employed will pay half the required Medicare tax, and this amount will be deducted directly from their paycheck. The remaining tax will be paid by their employer.

Those who are self-employed are required to pay the full Medicare Tax amount, both employee and employer contributions.

If you earn more, you are going to pay more.

The Affordable Care Act added an Additional Medicare Tax that was first applied in January 2013. It affected those who earned above the following modified adjusted gross income (MAGI) levels.

- Single or head of household - $200,000

- Married filing jointly - $250,000

- Married filing separately - $125,000

- Qualifying widow(er) with dependent child - $200,000

Any income above these amounts would be charged an additional 0.9 percent in Medicare taxes. Unlike the traditional Medicare Tax, this tax is paid entirely by the employee. The employer makes no contributions.

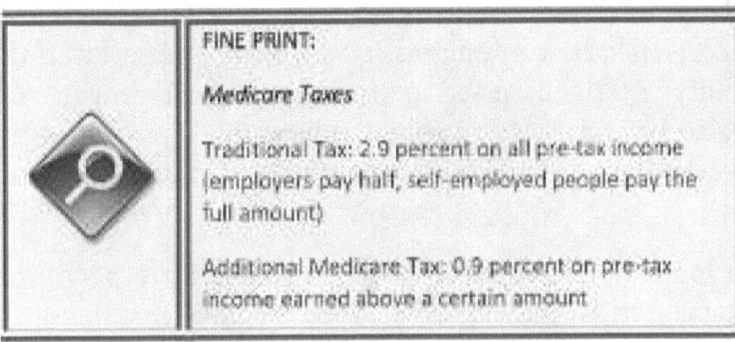

FINE PRINT:

Medicare Taxes

Traditional Tax: 2.9 percent on all pre-tax income (employers pay half, self-employed people pay the full amount)

Additional Medicare Tax: 0.9 percent on pre-tax income earned above a certain amount

For example, a single employed person earning $210,000 per year would pay 1.45 percent in Medicare taxes for the first $200,000 but a 2.35 percent tax (1.45 percent + 0.9 percent) on the remaining $10,000. The employer would continue paying 1.45 percent for the full range of income.

Someone who is self-employed would pay the standard 2.9 percent Medicare tax rate on any income below the threshold amount, $200,000, and 3.8 percent (2.9 percent + 0.9 percent) on any income over that threshold, in this case $10,000.

Monthly Premiums

Another cost expenditure that many do not consider until they are in the throes of Medicare is the monthly premium. Part A premiums may be free for certain beneficiaries but Parts B, C and D each have separate costs.

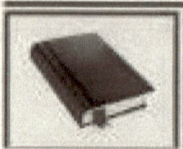

DEFINITION:

A premium is a fee paid periodically, usually every month, for a service.

The cost of Part A premiums is waived for those meeting the disability criteria discussed in Chapter 2. The monthly premiums will also be waived for eligible applicants 65 years of age and older who have contributed Medicare payroll taxes for at least 10 years.

If an individual has not contributed to Medicare payroll taxes personally, that individual may be eligible for free Part A premiums if their spouse or former spouse had done so. As always, there is fine print to consider:

- If someone divorces and remarries, they are only eligible for free Part A premiums based on their current spouse's record.

- If someone gets a divorce and remains single, they may be eligible for free Part A premiums based on the record of any of their former spouses so long as they were married to that person for at least 10 years.

- If someone is a widow, their marriage needs to have lasted at least nine months to be eligible for free Part A premiums.

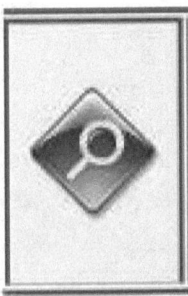
The government looks at tax contributions in terms of quarters. Forty calendar quarters (10 years) are required to receive Part A coverage for free. An individual who has contributed less than this amount needs to pay a monthly premium for Part A services that depends on how many quarters they paid Medicare taxes. For those who contributed between 30 and 39 quarters of taxes, their monthly premium in 2018 will be $232.00. For those who contributed less than 30 quarters, their monthly premium will be $433.00.

In 2018, Part B costs range from $134 per month to $428.60 per month depending on an individual's prior tax returns. The lower-end premiums apply to those earning less than $85,000 on their individual tax returns or less than $170,000 on a joint tax return. The upper-end premiums target those earning more than $160,000 (individual) or $320,000 (joint). They include the lower tier premium plus an amount referred to as the Income Related Monthly Adjustment Amount (IRMAA). Medicare uses tax returns from 2 years prior to determine how much IRMAA should be added to your premium. There is also a deductible of $183 for the year to consider. All of these costs may be adjusted on an annual basis.

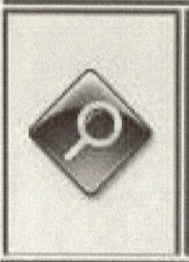

Premiums for Part C and Part D have greater variability as these parts of Medicare are run by private insurance companies. Part D premiums differ depending on the specific policy you choose. However, additional costs may be tagged onto the monthly premium based on how much money you make.

For those earning less than $85,000 on their individual tax returns or less than $170,000 on a joint tax return, there is no added IRMAA cost for Part D coverage. For those with higher incomes, an extra $12.40 to $77.40 is added to the premium cost every month. These costs reflect the rates for 2019.

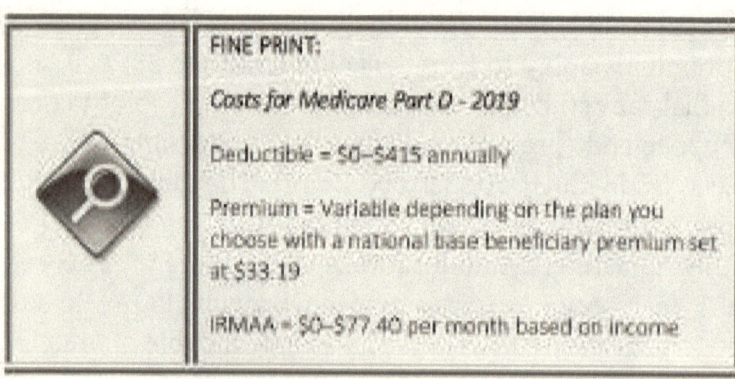

Similar to Part B, income tax returns from 2 years prior are used to decide how much you will pay.

The Centers for Medicare and Medicaid Services does not always release the updated premium and IRMAA amounts for the coming year before Open Enrollment Period starts. Depending on the year, there have been delays on this information well into

November. At the time of this publication, Part A and Part B information has not yet been released but Part D information is available. Be sure to visit the Diagnosis Life site where updates will be posted as soon as they are announced.

As a reminder, Open Enrollment begins on October 15 and ends on December 7 each year. You can wait for the official CMS numbers to come out before you enroll or you can use data from the previous year as a guide, understanding that this is only an estimate. You are likely to pay more since there is a consistent pattern of rates increasing each year.

Late Fees

Turning 65 years old does not mean you are automatically enrolled in Medicare. If only it were that easy!

Only people who are receiving Social Security benefits at the time of their 65th birthday get the benefit of automatic enrollment. Their Part A (if it is not free) and Part B premiums are deducted from their Social Security checks.

Everyone else is on the hook for late penalties if they do not know when and how to sign up. This trips people up more than you realize. Because maximum Social Security are not paid out until 67 years old, many people defer retirement until after they become eligible for Medicare. Quite simply, many people continue to work past 65 years old and continue on their employer-sponsored health plans. Medicare is the furthest thing from their minds.

FINE PRINT:

Medicare Sign-up without Paying Late Penalties

Initial Enrollment Period = +/- 3 months from your 65th birthday

Special Enrollment Period = Within 8 months of leaving an employer-sponsored health plan (or the job that offers you that health plan) but ONLY IF the employer has more than 20 full-time employees

Late fees are applied to those who sign up for Part A, Part B and/or Part D after their Initial Enrollment Period ends. This is where a little knowledge goes a long way. The Initial Enrollment Period is narrow: It begins 3 months before your 65th birthday and extends 3 months after that birthday, leaving you with only seven months to apply.

People who have existing health insurance through their employer or their spouse's employer can skip their Initial Enrollment Period and sign up during an optional Special Enrollment Period instead. This Special Enrollment Period begins when you leave your job or your employer-sponsored health plan, **whichever comes first**, and lasts for eight months. However, be careful! If your employer employs less than 20 full-time employees or its equivalent, you are not eligible for a Special Enrollment Period and could face late penalties if you miss signing up during the Initial Enrollment Period.

Medicare's late penalties are based on how long a person could have had coverage. Part A adds 10 percent to the monthly premiums for twice the number of years a person had been eligible before they signed up. A year is defined as a full 12-month period. For example, if you were eligible for Part A two years before you signed up, you will pay the higher premium for four years (twice the number of years) before you can return to the original premium rate.

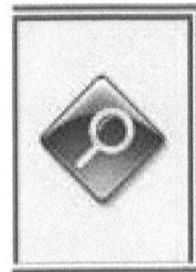

FINE PRINT:

Part A Late Fees

10% added to the monthly premium

Duration of penalty: Twice the number of YEARS of missed eligibility

Part B late penalties tag on an extra 10 percent to premiums but does so for every year that a person had been eligible for Part B. For example, if you were eligible for Part B two years before you signed up, you will pay 20 percent (number of years times 10 percent) more in premiums each month. The added costs go on indefinitely and do not end like the penalties in Part A.

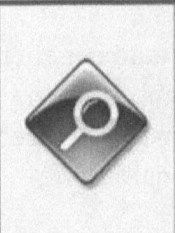

FINE PRINT:

Part B Late Fees

10% added to the monthly premium for every YEAR of missed eligibility

Duration of penalty: Long-standing

A 1 percent late enrollment Part D penalty will be added for every month (not year) you were eligible and did not have prescription drug coverage from another source. This Part D late fee is calculated off of the national base beneficiary premium of $33.19 (in 2019) rather than the higher premiums from the different plans some people choose.

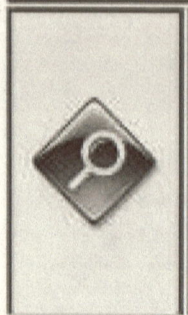

FINE PRINT:

Part D Late Fees

1% of the national base beneficiary premium for every MONTH of missed eligibility added to the actual monthly premium

Duration of penalty: Life-long unless you were < 65 years old when you first became eligible

Since the national base beneficiary premium can change from year to year, the late penalty will change as well but you will pay the penalty for the life of your coverage. Yes, you will be penalized as long as you have Medicare Part D. The one exception to this penalty occurs if your eligibility began before the age of 65. Once you turn 65 years old, the penalty will be removed.

Altogether, these Medicare costs quickly add up and beneficiaries require thoughtful preparation before they jump into the fray. They need to do their research on what plans will work best for them, and in a timely manner to avoid costly penalties.

Deductibles, Co-insurance, & Co-payments

Paying monthly premiums does not mean that the rest of your health care is provided free of charge. Deductibles, co-insurance and co-payments factor strongly into the equation.

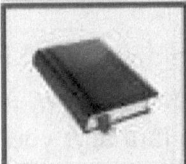

DEFINITION:

A deductible is a fixed dollar amount you pay for healthcare services before your insurance coverage kicks in.

For each inpatient hospital stay up to 60 days in 2019, there is a Part A deductible of $1,340. You will pay the same amount whether you stay 2 days or 60 days. Not that anyone wants to be in the hospital longer, but in one sense, the longer you stay the bigger the bargain.

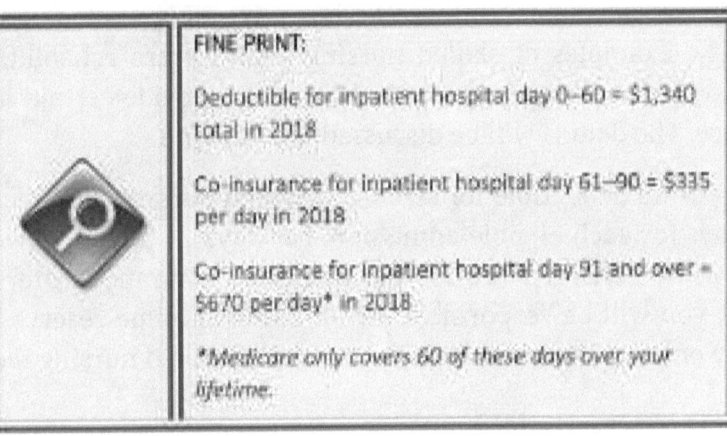

FINE PRINT:

Deductible for inpatient hospital day 0–60 = $1,340 total in 2018

Co-insurance for inpatient hospital day 61–90 = $335 per day in 2018

Co-insurance for inpatient hospital day 91 and over = $670 per day* in 2018

*Medicare only covers 60 of these days over your lifetime.

On the other hand, costs begin to accrue for stays longer than 60 days. For day 61 to 90, there is an added price tag of $335 per day and for stays after 91 days, a cost of $670 dollars per day. For stays 91 days and longer, you start to dig into your lifetime reserve days. Medicare limits you to a maximum 60 reserve days in your lifetime.* After that, you will pay full out-of-pocket expenses.

Example: Inpatient Hospital Costs for a 92 Day Stay in 2018

Hospital Day	Cost Per Day	Cost Total
Days 0-60 (60 days)	Deductible	$1,340
Days 61-90 (30 days)	$335 per day	$10,050 ($335 x 30 days)
Days 91-92 (2 days)	$670 per day	$1,340 ($670 x 2 days)
		$12,730

The billing cycle starts all over again if you are discharged from the hospital and are admitted to the hospital another time. As an example, if you are admitted to the hospital in January, you will pay the $1,340 deductible and co-insurance for your stay after 60 days. If you stay 92 days total, you will have used up two of your lifetime reserve days, leaving you with 58 days. If you are admitted to the hospital again in June, you will pay another $1,340 deductible and so on. For your health and well-being, I pray you do not require repeated hospital stays that long.

Costs are calculated differently for stays in a skilled nursing facility. Examples of skilled nursing facilities are rehabilitation centers and nursing homes as long as they provide certain levels of care. The details will be discussed in Chapter 8.

There is no deductible for stays in a skilled nursing facility up to 20 days for each eligible admission. For days 21 to 100, however, you will be charged $167.50 per day as co-insurance. After that time, you will be responsible for all costs. Lifetime reserve days apply only for inpatient hospital stays, not skilled nursing facility stays.

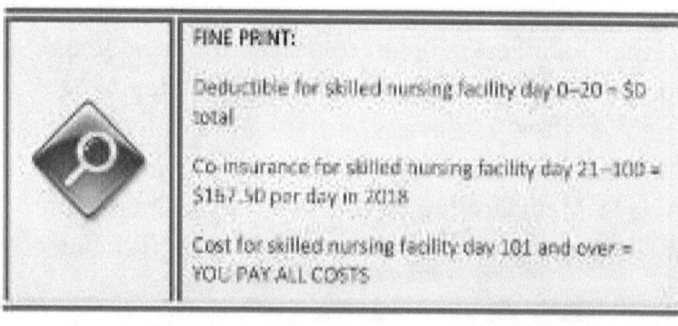

FINE PRINT:

Deductible for skilled nursing facility day 0-20 = $0 total

Co-insurance for skilled nursing facility day 21-100 = $167.50 per day in 2018

Cost for skilled nursing facility day 101 and over = YOU PAY ALL COSTS

Part D deductibles will vary based on the prescription plan you choose. Some may have no deductible while the maximum deductible allowable by federal guidelines is $415 for 2019. This capped amount changes, and usually increases, on an annual basis.

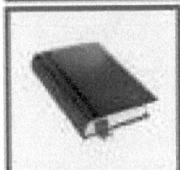

DEFINITION:

A co-insurance is a fixed percentage you pay for a product or service. The cost you pay will differ depending on how expensive the item is.

Part B requires that you pay a co-insurance with the exception of Wellness Visits and specific preventive medicine services which are free. These co-insurance costs, often 20 percent, apply to outpatient services ranging from doctor's appointments to laboratory tests to diabetic supplies. This will be addressed in detail in Chapter 4.

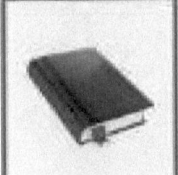

DEFINITION:

A co-payment or co-pay is a fixed fee you pay every time you purchase a product or service. Regardless of the cost of the item, your payment will always be the same.

Part D services usually require a co-payment or co-insurance for purchases of medication. This will also be addressed in Chapter 4.

The expected costs for 2018 and 2019, including potential late fees, are broken down in the following tables for Parts A, B and D.

Medicare Part A: Expected Costs in 2018
Based on Quarters of Medicare Eligible Employment

		40+ quarters	30–39 quarters	< 30 quarters
No Penalty	Monthly premium	$0	$232	$422
	Annual Cost	$0	$2,784	$5,064
With Penalty	Late penalty	$0	$23.20	$42.20
	Monthly premium	$0	$255.20	$464.20
	Annual cost	$0	$3,062.40	$5,570.40

Medicare Part B: Expected Costs in 2018
Based on Income Tax Returns

	Single: < $85,000 -or- Joint: < $170,000 Married but Filing Separate: < $85,000	Single: $85,000–$107,000 -or- Joint: $170,000–$214,000	Single: $107,000–$133,500 -or- Joint: $214,000–$267,000	Single: $133,500–$160,000 -or- Joint: $267,000–$320,000	Single: > $160,000 -or- Joint: > $320,000 Married but Filing Separate: > $85,000
Monthly Premium + IRMAA	$134	$187.50	$267.90	$348.30	$428.60
Deductible	$183	$183	$183	$183	$183
Annual Cost	$1,791	$2,433	$3,398	$4,363	$5,326

A late penalty of 10% is added to the monthly premium for every YEAR of missed enrolment after eligibility, i.e., one year = 10%, two years = 20%, three years = 30% etc.

Medicare Part D: Expected Costs in 2019
Based on Income Tax Returns

	Single: < $85,000 -or- Joint: < $170,000 Married but Filing Separate: < $85,000	Single: $85,000–$107,000 -or- Joint: $170,000–$214,000	Single: $107,000–$133,500 -or- Joint: $214,000–$267,000	Single: $133,500–$160,000 -or- Joint: $267,000–$320,000	Single: $160,000–$500,000 or- Joint: $320,000–$750,000 Married but Filing Separate: > $85,000–$415,000	Single: > $500,000 or- Joint: > $750,000 Married but Filing Separate: > $415,000
Monthly Premium	Variable depending on the plan selected (National base beneficiary premium = $33.19)					
Added Costs	$0	$12.40	$31.90	$51.40	$70.90	$77.40
Deductible	Variable depending on the plan selected (Minimum deductible $0, maximum deductible $415)					
Annual Cost (Min)	$398	$547	$781	$1,015	$1,249	$1,327

A late penalty of 1% of the national base beneficiary premium rounded to the nearest $0.10 is added to the monthly premium for every full MONTH of missed enrollment after eligibility, i.e., 10 months = $3.30, 20 months = $6.60, 30 months = $10.00 etc.

Medicare Assignment

All this discussion about costs has been getting a little expensive, wouldn't you say? It can get pricey depending on what healthcare provider you choose too. There are two important things that you need to ask your healthcare provider before you get started.

The first thing to know is obvious: does your healthcare provider take Medicare patients? If your provider has opted out of Medicare, he can charge you whatever he wants and you will be responsible for all costs out of your own pocket. Medicare will not pay for any services, even for services usually covered by Medicare.

In this case, that provider may ask you to sign a private contract to review the finer details of your financial obligations. This contract, however, cannot include a clause for urgent or emergency care—it would not be ethical for a provider to turn you away because of dollars and cents in times of a true emergency.

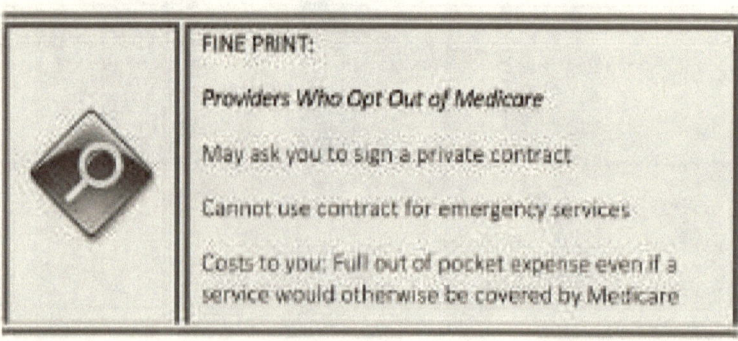

FINE PRINT:

Providers Who Opt Out of Medicare

May ask you to sign a private contract

Cannot use contract for emergency services

Costs to you: Full out of pocket expense even if a service would otherwise be covered by Medicare

It is in your best interest to seek out healthcare providers who do accept Medicare. At times you may not have a choice if there are limited resources in your area capable of providing proper care.

For those providers who opt in for Medicare there is another important distinction: does the provider accept assignment? Medicare sets a Physician Fee Schedule for all covered services. Accepting assignment means that your provider has signed a contract with the government agreeing to all of these fixed fees. Furthermore, they will only charge you the amount of your co-insurance and Medicare deductible, not more. The Physician Fee Schedule keeps the costs to you as low as possible regardless of where you live in the country.

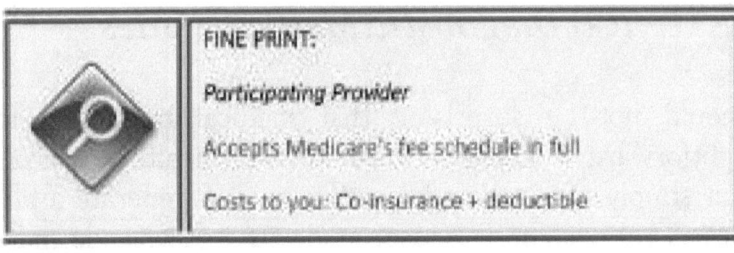

FINE PRINT:

Participating Provider

Accepts Medicare's fee schedule in full

Costs to you: Co-insurance + deductible

Non-participating providers agree to accept Medicare as insurance but may accept only some of the Physician Fee Schedule or none at all. They can charge you up to 15 percent more than the cost recommended by Medicare. This "limiting charge" is an attempt at cost containment so that no more than 15 percent of the cost will be added on top of your usual co-insurance and deductible.

Unfortunately, limiting charges do not apply to durable medical equipment and non-participating suppliers of that equipment. These suppliers can charge you whatever they want. A list of durable medical equipment is provided in Chapter 4.

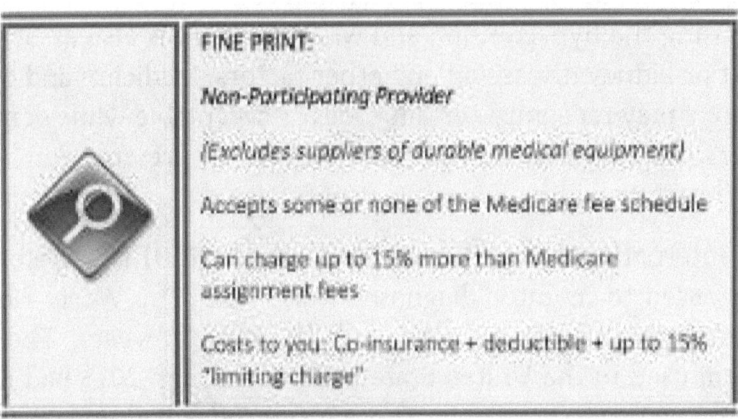

FINE PRINT:

Non-Participating Provider

(Excludes suppliers of durable medical equipment)

Accepts some or none of the Medicare fee schedule

Can charge up to 15% more than Medicare assignment fees

Costs to you: Co-insurance + deductible + up to 15% "limiting charge"

Unless otherwise stated, the costs described later in this book will refer to those of participating providers accepting assignment.

ICD Diagnostic Medical Codes

It should not be surprising that medical billing is not a straightforward and simple process. Your healthcare provider cannot simply write down hypertension and generate a bill for services. Every diagnosis is associated with its own code and your provider has to choose the right one. That is not always as easy as it sounds.

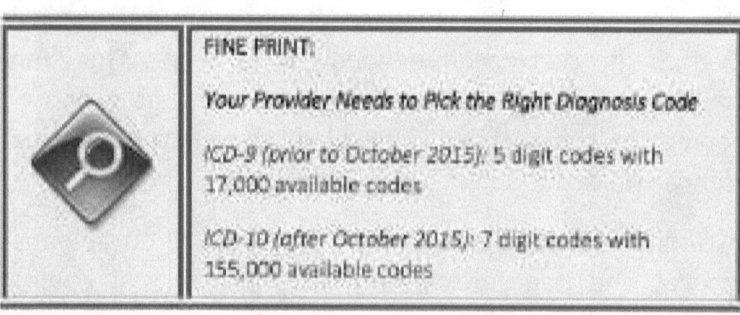

FINE PRINT:

Your Provider Needs to Pick the Right Diagnosis Code

ICD-9 (prior to October 2015): 5 digit codes with 17,000 available codes

ICD-10 (after October 2015): 7 digit codes with 155,000 available codes

There are many different diagnoses for the same type of problem. For example, the specific hypertension code will depend on what is causing the hypertension and whether there is also associated heart or kidney disease among other factors. Medicare and other insurers may recognize certain codes as acceptable while denying others for payment. That puts a lot of pressure on your healthcare provider.

The International Classification of Diseases (ICD) is a system of codes used to monitor diagnoses worldwide. The World Health Organization heads revisions to ICD every 10 years. The ICD system used in the United States, ICD-9, through 2015 had more than 17,000 codes available. Those ICD-9 codes had up to 5 digits to define a condition.

ICD-10 was used in other countries long before it was instituted in the United States. The country had been slow to implement it and with good reason. It is a drastic change, expanding the coding system to 7 digits and more than 155,000 different codes. The government delayed implementation of ICD-10 use for three years after lobbying by the American Medical Association but finally took the leap in October 2015.

The transition to the new system has run smoother than expected though it is estimated that more than 10 percent of codes are erroneous! If you feel you have received a charge or bill in error, it could be due to a coding problem. Your healthcare provider may need to change a diagnostic code for services to be covered by Medicare. You may need to contact your provider's medical or billing office to address the issue.

Things are sure to get more complicated in the future. The World Health Organization intends to present ICD-11 at the World Health Assembly in May 2019. If the version is adopted, it would come into effect in January 2022. Based on the delay in utilizing ICD-10, it is unlikely the United States would make a change to ICD-11 in the near future.

MEDICARE PRESCRIPTIONS

Prescriptions by the Numbers

Prescription medications and medical supplies are big business. In 2016, more than 4.45 million medications were prescribed. That year $328.6 billion was spent on prescription drugs with Medicare accounting for $174 billion of those expenditures. Understanding when and where we can cut costs can make a difference not only for those on Medicare but for all healthcare consumers.

As much as we try to stay healthy by eating healthy and exercising regularly, the unfortunate truth is that medications are sometimes necessary to treat a condition or to at least minimize symptoms.

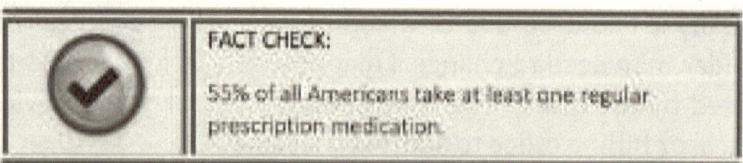

FACT CHECK:

55% of all Americans take at least one regular prescription medication.

If you are one of the lucky ones, your dependence on prescription medications will be minimal as you age. The statistics unfortunately are stacked against you.

The Consumer Reports National Research Center published survey results in April 2017 around the use of prescription medications. Looking at 1947 American adults, they found that 55 percent of them took a regular prescription and the average person took four prescription drugs. As many as 75 percent also took an over-the-counter medication.

A survey looking at both prescription and over the counter medications was reported in the Journal of the American Medical

Association (JAMA) in 2008. Of 3005 adults between the ages of 57 and 85 years old, 81 percent used at least one medication and 29 percent used five or more medications. For those older than 75 years old, five or more medications were used by as many as 36 percent of those surveyed.

In 2015, research by Charlesworth et al. published in found that 25 percent of people aged 65 to 69 years old take at least five prescription drugs to treat chronic conditions. That number rises to 46 percent for people between the ages of 70 and 79.

An updated 2016 study in JAMA Internal Medicine reported that 87 percent of seniors between 62 and 85 years old who live at home take at least one prescription medication. The number increases to 36 percent for people taking five or more prescription drugs.

Medicare beneficiaries who were discharged from a hospital to a skilled nursing facility were prescribed an average of 14 medications! This stunning statistic was reported in the Journal of Hospital Medicine in 2016.

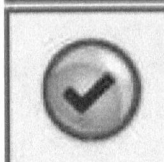

FACT CHECK:

In 2016, a survey in JAMA Internal Medicine estimated that 36% of people over 62 years old used five or more prescription medications.

Regardless of the study, the results are comparable. Americans use a lot of medications, more so if they are on Medicare. The point is that there are a lot of medications being prescribed on a regular basis and therefore opportunities for saving.

Medication Price Tag

Some generic medications cost cents on the dollar while others cost thousands of dollars for a single dose. Examples can be seen in the brand-name products COSENTYX®[1] and TALTZ®[2] used to treat complicated diseases such as ankylosing spondylosis, plaque psoriasis and psoriatic arthritis. Without insurance, these medications may cost up to $4,900 to $5,400, respectively, for each dose. These medications are usually administered once every 4 weeks but they require a dose titration to start where you will require several doses over the first one to two months. One could easily go bankrupt paying these costs out-of-pocket but if these medications could mean the difference between quality living and suffering, what would your health be worth?

Enter insurance. Insurance allows a person to pay a small portion of the expense, a co-pay, while their insurance pays the difference. Often the insurance company has negotiated a price with the pharmaceutical company for certain medications. This is how formularies come into play. Formularies are essentially a preferred list of medications for you to choose from.

Different insurance companies will have different formularies. The intention is to save both you and the insurance company money, but to be honest, the benefits often favor your health plan.

If a medication is not on your formulary, your insurance plan may require you to go through a special approval process known as a prior authorization to get the medication. Then again, they can choose to deny coverage of a medication altogether, shifting the entire cost to you. It is in your best interest to have your healthcare provider prescribe medications from your formulary to help keep costs down.

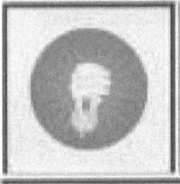

CONCEPT:

Insurance companies negotiate the prices of medications with pharmaceutical companies to save money.

People tend to think of insurance companies as the "bad guy". To make a profit, they want to pay as little as possible for medications and this leads them to negotiate with the drug companies. By encouraging you to pick medications that they get at a bargain rate, the insurance companies pay less of a cost differential than with other medications. By getting you to pick the least expensive medications, they save even more.

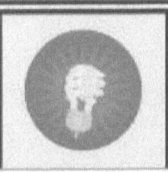

CONCEPT:

Total medication cost – Your co-payment =

What the insurance company pays

Medications are ranked using a tier system according to your insurance plan, Medicare Part D or otherwise. Generic drugs are often on tier 1 while tiers 2 and above may offer more expensive brand name products. The higher the tier, the higher the co-pay.

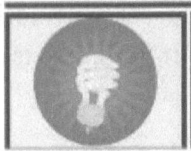

CONCEPT:

The higher the tier, the higher the co-payment.

You will pay a co-payment each time you fill a prescription whether it is a medication new to you or not. Co-pays can range from a few dollars up to $30 or more per prescription. Considering the average adult over 65 years old pays for 5 prescriptions, refills included, that could quickly add up to a lot of dollars.

Brand-Name vs. generic medications

It fascinates me how loyal some people are to brand-name products. If someone has stock in a company, that is one thing. The majority of the time, however, the preference for a brand name is for the purpose of some presumed status or reputation. People like belonging to a prestigious group. They like having the best of the best.

Let me fill you in on a little secret: brand-name loyalty in medicine is not necessary. It rarely matters. A generic version of a branded medication is by definition the same chemical compound as its counterpart. With the same ingredient and the same dose strength, the clinical effect should technically be the same.

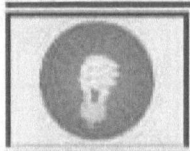

CONCEPT:

Generic medications are often as good as brand name medications.

Like anything in life, however, there are shades of gray. There may be times when a medication is processed differently between pharmaceutical companies. Perhaps the mechanism for deriving or purifying the drug is unique at one facility versus another, even though the final product—the active ingredient—is the same.

With this in mind, there remains a possibility that a person may react differently to one generic medication versus another generic or the branded product. For example, residue of a processing chemical could be present on the drug.

Some of my patients have developed an allergic reaction to a generic version of a medication while tolerating the brand-name version. I have seen it go so far as a patient responding well to a generic medication from one pharmaceutical company but not the same generic medication from another company. The reverse effect is also possible: an individual tolerating a generic version of a drug over the brand name. Of course some sort of placebo effect could be at play here too, but these examples illustrate rare occasions when a brand-name product may be indicated. Again, this is the exception rather than the rule.

Not all medications have a generic version on the market. A medication may still be under patent by the pharmaceutical company that discovered that drug. In this scenario, generic versions of the medication cannot be made by other companies until that patent expires. Once the patent runs out, generic medications may be made by one and often several other companies which decreases costs of the medication by virtue of market competition. Think of it as good old capitalism at work.

Of course, good old capitalism has also been known to backfire. Sometimes pharmaceutical companies take over patents for generic drugs or take interest in manufacturing certain drugs for profit. In September 2015, Martin Shkreli, then CEO of Turing Pharmaceuticals, obtained the manufacturing license for Daraprim (pyramethamine) and increased the cost of the anti-parasitic drug used to treat AIDS/HIV patients by more than 5,500 percent! Where are the morals?

A medication could also be the first of its kind or in a class that only has brand-name medications available. COSENTYX and TALTZ are perfect examples of this sort of medication, which explains, to some extent, their high cost. If other classes of medications are not effective or appropriate for an individual, a healthcare provider may need to prescribe one of these more expensive medications.

The lesson to learn here is simple: sometimes brand-name medications are necessary and sometimes they are not.

Switching Brand-Name to Generic

Insurance companies will often send requests to their beneficiaries suggesting changes from a brand-name to a generic medication. Healthcare providers receive similar mailings. The intention is to cut costs for both the beneficiary and the insurance company. You may have a lower co-pay and your insurance will pay less when they pay the cost difference for a cheaper medication.

Before you pounce on the offer, be sure that there is actually a generic version of the medication available. Oftentimes insurance companies will include generic medications on that mailing list that are in the same class of medications but are not actually the same drug.

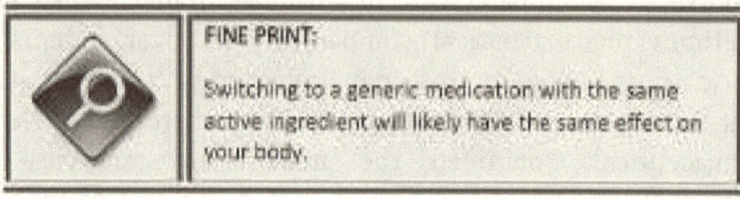

FINE PRINT:

Switching to a generic medication with the same active ingredient will likely have the same effect on your body.

This is where the insurance companies begin to think more about their bottom line than what may be best for your health. Often medications in the same class, meaning that they work by the same mechanism of action, have the same or a similar effect on an individual. This cannot be guaranteed, however.

Everyone has a different metabolism and may respond differently to another medication, even if it works in the same way. If a medication has had a positive clinical effect on a person, it seems a shame to change it unnecessarily. A generic of the same exact medication, however, is a very reasonable option.

The Good and Bad of Free Samples

Many doctor's offices provide free medication samples while others are steering away from this practice. Traditionally, pharmaceutical companies send representatives to medical offices to deliver the samples. These representatives may provide literature and studies reporting benefits of the medication while being available to answer questions about their products.

Finding one-on-one time to talk with a doctor may be easy for patients (though some of you may disagree) but not so for pharmaceutical representatives. How could they educate the doctor on the miracles of their wonder drug if they never got to talk to him? After all, most doctors are busy seeing patients or completing administrative tasks usually into and through their lunch hours (or more often the case, lunch minutes). To get the doctor's attention, some pharmaceutical companies began to entice doctors for their time.

In the days of yesteryear, long before I came to practice medicine, physicians would be offered compensation for their sit-down time with these representatives. Compensation was often indirect with simple "gifts" ranging from pens to sticky notes labeled with the pharmaceutical company or medication name.

Drug lunches became commonplace as the offer of free food was used to draw physicians out of their offices to eat a bite or two during their lunch hour. Outright bribes and kickbacks in the way of vacation travel and offers of company stock have even been reported. As you can imagine, these tactics could heavily influence what medications a healthcare provider would choose to prescribe.

It could be argued that by giving free samples the pharmaceutical companies are offering a service. They are not making but actually losing money by giving the product away. Some may go so far as to say they are not affecting a doctor's prescribing habits because the doctor is not pulling out their Rx pad to write an actual prescription. The doctor is only handing out samples.

The reality is something quite different.

What does the doctor do when free samples of a specific medication are no longer available? He could change to another medication but if a patient is satisfied with the initial product, he could well write out a prescription for that same brand-name medication.

When considering prescriptions for other patients, that brand-name drug could be one of the first that comes to mind given his close proximity and experience with the medication. Doctors say that they are not influenced by interactions with the pharmaceutical industry but some studies have shown otherwise.

Think about what this could mean for your health. If your provider is directly or indirectly influenced to prescribe certain medications and starts you on a more expensive medication, this will affect your out-of-pocket costs.

I am proud to have gone through a family medicine residency program at the University of Connecticut where all interactions with pharmaceutical representatives and residents were supervised by a staff pharmacist to assure that only objective data was shared between all parties and that no gifts of any kind were exchanged. This sort of training allowed me to keep perspective not only through my medical training but into my clinical practice.

Failure to adhere to the mandatory reporting will result in fines to the pharmaceutical company. Fines may be as high as $1,000 to $10,000 per infraction but could reach as high as $10,000 to $1,000,000 over a year if it is proven that data was intentionally withheld.

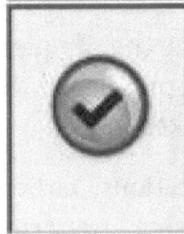

FACT CHECK:

The Affordable Care Act limits the amount of gifts a pharmaceutical company can offer to healthcare providers. You can see if your healthcare provider accepted gifts over the allowed amount at www.cms.gov/openpayments/.

The Physician Payments Sunshine Act does not mean that free samples go away. Free samples, medication vouchers and rebate cards are not considered gifts according to this new law. What it may mean is reduced face time for the representatives with the doctors, which may well be a good thing as the information provided is likely biased in some way. It is salesmanship after all.

Decreasing the influence of the pharmaceutical companies on prescribing habits could also encourage healthcare providers to favor generic medications over brand-name ones. The end result could be reduced costs for the healthcare system at large.

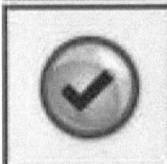

FACT CHECK:

The Affordable Care Act does not consider free samples, medication vouchers or rebate cards to be gifts.

Most medication samples are for brand-name medications, not generic ones. These samples tend to be the newest to the market and for that reason tend to be the most expensive. Most of these medications are placed on tier 2 and above on insurance formularies and have the highest co-payments.

Given their limited supply, healthcare providers tend to reserve free samples for their most needy patients, those who cannot afford their medications. Still, sometimes the distribution of these samples may include other groups of people looking for a deal. The cost savings for the patient who receives free samples is obvious.

Free samples are a clever marketing device. Once the samples are no longer available, patients will often be prescribed these higher-cost medications with higher out-of-pocket costs.

A doctor may offer a different set of medications, either an alternative free sample or a less expensive prescription medication, but that is a disruption to the patient's care. New medications risk new side effects. Will the new medication be as effective as the old one? Changes to a medication regimen require trial and error and close monitoring, which could lead to increased frequency of doctor visits and other healthcare costs.

As you see, there is good and bad that comes with using free samples. The ugly takes the shape of a donut hole.

How The Donut Hole Works

Before you start to drool over the possibility of a delicious bakery treat, remember that I am a doctor first and foremost so put down the donut (and pick up a piece of fruit)! What we are looking at here is not a sweet ball of fried dough but the gaping hole it leaves behind, the missing piece. The "donut hole" is the gap in the coverage of prescription medications for Medicare Part D.

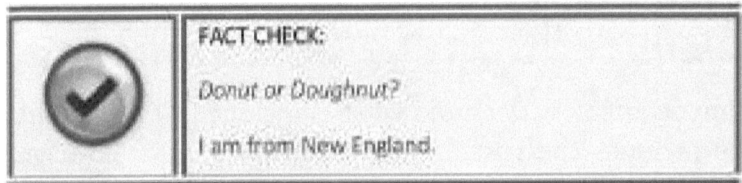

FACT CHECK:

Donut or Doughnut?

I am from New England.

It is a very interesting concept and one that leaves many seniors baffled as they try to manage their healthcare costs. I will do my best to explain it to you.

For 2019, the numbers are as follows.

- **Medicare Part D Coverage (Up to $3,820)**

- **Donut Hole ($3,820-$5,100)**

- **Catastrophic Coverage ($5,100 and over)**

Depending on your Medicare Part D plan, you will first pay out a deductible. Once this dollar amount has been spent, Medicare Part D will begin to cover the cost of your medications. For each prescription you fill, you will pay a co-payment. The cost of the co-payment depends on the tier of medication as discussed earlier. The higher the tier, the higher the co-payment.

Your Part D plan covers the difference between the negotiated cost of the medication and your co-payment. This coverage continues until you and your Part D plan have spent $3,820 (at least this is the value set for 2019). This limit will change annually.

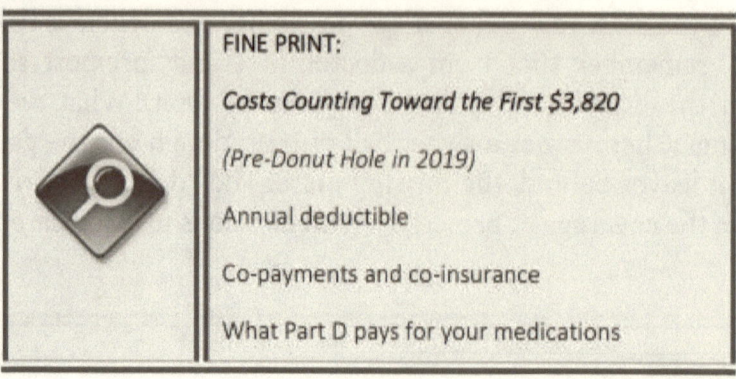

FINE PRINT:

Costs Counting Toward the First $3,820

(Pre-Donut Hole in 2019)

Annual deductible

Co-payments and co-insurance

What Part D pays for your medications

It is important to understand what is included to that point. The $3,820 includes the cost of your deductible, your co-payments and the amount spent by Medicare to cover the remaining costs of your medications.

What it does not include are cost expenditures for your monthly premiums or for any medications not covered on your Part D formulary. Also, medications purchased outside of the United States do not meet criteria. People often look to other countries, like Canada, for lower drug costs but will it save them money in the long run when you consider what happens in the donut hole?

When you and Medicare reach that $3,820 limit, the cost of your prescription medications increases significantly.

Welcome to the donut hole.

The donut hole is a dark place where I have seen far too many people struggle not only with their finances but their health. People who have had their medical conditions stabilized on their medication regimens may no longer be able to afford them. They may have to cut other expenses in their life, hopefully not in the way of food, housing expenses or necessary utilities. They may opt to stop their medications altogether (please, don't do this!).

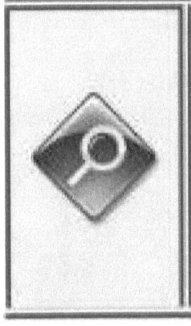

FINE PRINT:

Costs NOT Counting Toward the First $3,820 (Pre-Donut Hole in 2019)

Monthly premiums

Medications not covered by your Part D plan

Medications purchased outside of the United States

More often, healthcare providers will offer their patients less expensive medication options until the coverage gap closes. As discussed previously, there is no guarantee that these medication changes will work out. More monitoring may be required during the transition to these new medications to assure they are working properly.

Medicare Part D and its coverage gap came into existence in 2003. Since enactment of the ACA in 2010, there have been improvements that have decreased the cost burden to Medicare Part D beneficiaries during that coverage gap, although costs remain high.

Instead of paying a smaller fixed co-payment, you will pay an outright percentage of costs for your medications. You will not pay the full retail price of the medications because prices have been negotiated between your Part D plan and the pharmacies, whether it is a traditional on-site store or a mail-order pharmacy. This decreases costs to a certain extent but the blow to your wallet may be bigger than you anticipate.

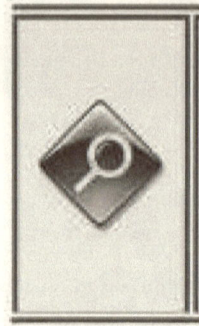

FINE PRINT:

Costs Counting Towards the Donut Hole in 2019

Your co-insurance of 25% for brand-name medications

Your co-insurance of 37% on generic medications

What Part D pays for your brand-name medications

You will spend 25 percent of the negotiated price on brand-name medications and 37 percent on generic medications. This means that 75 percent and 63 percent, respectively, of your medication expenses are covered by Medicare. The percentage you pay on generic medications will decrease to 25 percent by 2020.

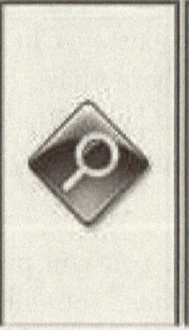

FINE PRINT:

Costs NOT Counting Toward the Donut Hole in 2019

Monthly premiums

What Part D pays for your generic medications

Medications not covered by your Part D plan

Medications purchased outside of the United States

Take a moment to consider what I told you about the monthly cost of COSENTYX and TALTZ. Retail costs were a whopping $4,900 to $5,400 per dose. In this scenario, what could have been an $80 co-pay for a high-tier medication may now cost the patient more than $2,500 for a one-month supply. Of course, the actual dollar amount of the co-payment or co-insurance will vary depending on the Medicare Part D plan someone has selected as well as what price the pharmaceutical company negotiated with the insurance plan.

The donut hole continues until one of two things happen: 1) the end of the annual Medicare calendar year is reached or 2) your annual prescription costs reach $5,100. That means you could be caught in the donut hole for as much as a hearty $1,280 (donut-hole end $5,100 minus donut-hole start $3,820) before you can get additional coverage.

Your co-insurances count towards the $1,280. The dollar amount that Medicare spends on your brand-name medications also counts towards the donut hole but the amount they spend on your generic medications does not. Again, your monthly premiums, non-formulary medications, and medications purchased outside of the United States are not counted towards the $1,280.

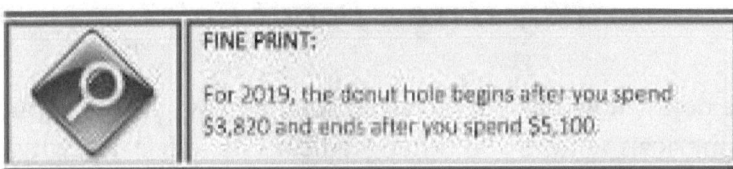

FINE PRINT:

For 2019, the donut hole begins after you spend $3,820 and ends after you spend $5,100.

Once the donut hole closes, you enter the phase of catastrophic coverage. Doesn't that sound delightful? At least the name acknowledges that by this point you have been saddled with an obscene amount of expenditures.

During catastrophic coverage, your spending reduces to smaller co-pays or co-insurances depending on the specific Part D plan you selected. For 2019, catastrophic coverage will cost either $3.40 for generic medications (or $8.50 for brand-name drugs) or 5 percent of the total cost of the medication, whichever cost is greater.

Why Have a Donut Hole?

If the donut hole has proven to be such a heavy financial burden for American seniors and other Medicare beneficiaries, why does it exist at all? The answer is simple: cost containment.

Ultimately, it would be ideal if each Medicare beneficiary did not have to pay for prescription medications at all. Even better, not to need them at all. Back to that good old diet, exercise and positive thinking. Relying on healthy living alone, unfortunately, is not realistic with the aging body and conditions that sneak in by virtue of our genetic makeup.

What the donut hole does is incentivize healthcare providers to keep costs in mind as they prescribe to their patients. Favoring cheaper medications to more expensive ones, their choices decide whether a person reaches that coverage gap in the first place. Also, when and if the coverage gap is reached, the costs to that person will be less because the medications are more cost-conscious.

What would happen if there were no financial constraints put on prescription costs? Would there be excessive amounts of brand-name medications prescribed at higher cost? Would pharmaceutical companies gain the upper hand with their advertising and marketing campaigns? Would people demand brand-name medications as a result?

You would be surprised how that prestige factor I mentioned earlier sneaks its way in. I have treated quite a few people with that mindset, who all but demand to try a certain medication because they believe it to be the best of the best. Those marketing campaigns work.

I will let you in on a not-so-secret secret. Generic medications are likely your best bet. These medications are available as generics because they have been around for many years. They have stood the test of time.

Newer medications may have been approved by the FDA with clinical data to support their use, but they do not have the years of experience to back them up that generics do. If you think about it, you could name quite a few medications that have been removed from the market for safety reasons in recent years. The prestige may rightly belong to the generic, and not the brand-name, products.

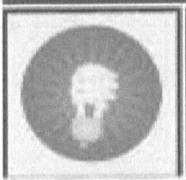

CONCEPT:

Generic medications have more years of clinical data and may be safer than some newer brand-name medications.

Healthcare costs are on the rise and the government is trying to prepare its resources. With the Medicare population increasing in size every year, they are trying to explore ways to decrease spending from the Medicare Trust Fund. It is not solely to save money but to preserve Medicare for future generations. You can almost see why they are going about it this way just as easily as you can see they are going about it all wrong.

The problem with the donut hole, among other things, is that those with the most complicated diseases or a compilation of medical conditions literally pay the most, almost as if they are penalized for being ill. They may have more needs, require more prescriptions. Perhaps they have failed to respond to generic medications and more expensive medications must be used to stabilize their health. There really ought to be a better way to do this. Health should be preserved for all.

Medicare Part B Medications

While the majority of prescription drug coverage is through Part D, Part B does cover a limited number of medications. After you pay the Part B deductible for the year, you will pay the 20 percent of the Medicare-approved amount for each of these medications. Keep in mind your doctor must accept assignment in order for you to be able to take advantage of Part B medications.

Certain vaccinations are covered under Medicare Part B. For those who qualify, these vaccines include:

- Hepatitis B vaccines

- Influenza (flu) vaccines

- Pneumococcal (pneumonia) vaccines

- Tetanus vaccines in specific cases

Hepatitis B shots are offered only to those considered at high risk. High risk factors for hepatitis B include diabetes, end-stage renal disease, hemophilia, past transfusion of blood products and being a healthcare worker at risk for exposure to the virus.

Flu shots are covered once every flu season for everyone.

Pneumonia shots are offered one-time only after age 65 years old. If a Medicare beneficiary is younger than 65 years old based on a disability and is considered at risk for pneumonia (e.g., is immunocompromised or has cardiopulmonary disease), he may qualify for two vaccinations, one prior and one after 65 years of age.

Tetanus vaccines are only offered in the case that a Medicare beneficiary has sustained an injury that increases the risk for tetanus infection, e.g., they cut themselves or stepped on a nail. Part B does not cover it as part of routine health maintenance even though tetanus vaccination is recommended every 10 years by the Advisory Committee on Immunization Practices (ACIP), a division of the U.S. Department of Health and Human Services. If you wanted to be vaccinated for this purpose, you would have to defer to your Part D coverage.

Shingles vaccination also does not fall under Part B coverage. It may or may not be covered by your Medicare Part D plan.

Also covered under Part B are medications that require the use of durable medical equipment. Examples are medications used in nebulizer machines and medications used in infusion pumps.

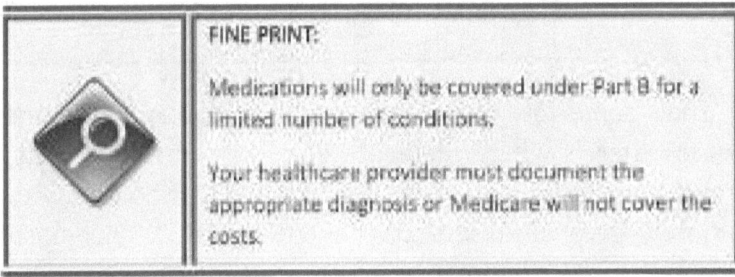

FINE PRINT:

Medications will only be covered under Part B for a limited number of conditions.

Your healthcare provider must document the appropriate diagnosis or Medicare will not cover the costs.

Medications that require administration by a licensed healthcare provider are generally covered under Part B as well. Injectable medications administered by you or other persons may include the following if certain conditions are met:

- Blood clotting factors for hemophilia

- Erythropoiesis-stimulating for anemia caused by end-stage renal disease and other specific conditions

- Intravenous immunoglobulin for primary immune deficiency

- Intravenous nutrition and tube feeding

- Medications for post-menopausal osteoporosis

- Other Medicare-approved injectable and infused medications administered by a licensed medical professional

FINE PRINT:

Medications will only be covered under Part B for a limited number of conditions.

Your healthcare provider must document the appropriate diagnosis or Medicare will not cover the costs.

Note that some of these medications require very specific diagnoses—here's where medical necessity comes into play. If a man needs an injectable osteoporosis medication, he is out of luck simply because he doesn't have a pair of X chromosomes. Medicare Part B will not cover the costs because osteoporosis alone is insufficient as a diagnosis and he obviously has not experienced menopause. Post-menopausal osteoporosis must be clearly specified for Part B coverage. He will have to rely on his Part D coverage or otherwise pay out of pocket even if his bones are equally as weak as a woman suffering in her menopausal years. Likewise, if the doctor prescribing the medication does not clearly delineate her condition as post-menopausal when he prescribes it, the woman may equally be charged for the medication.

Part B coverage of medications taken by mouth is even more restricted.

- Anti-nausea medication used within 48 hours of a chemotherapy regimen at strengths available in intravenous form

- Anti-cancer medication at strengths available in intravenous form or as a prodrug or activated version of the intravenous medication

People with renal failure or end-stage renal disease may also be eligible for Part B coverage of specific medications. For those who have had a kidney transplant, Medicare will provide Part B coverage for the immunosuppressant medications needed to prevent the body from rejecting the organ.

After 36 months, some of these transplant patients will lose their Medicare coverage if they no longer meet the criteria for renal failure. After all, they now have a functioning kidney and do not meet disability status. This is an unfortunate situation because they will still need to pay for these immunosuppressant medications for the rest of their lives.

For coverage to continue, the patient needs to qualify for Medicare by the traditional eligibility standards of age or disability. Coverage of these medications requires that the transplant had taken place in a Medicare-certified facility.

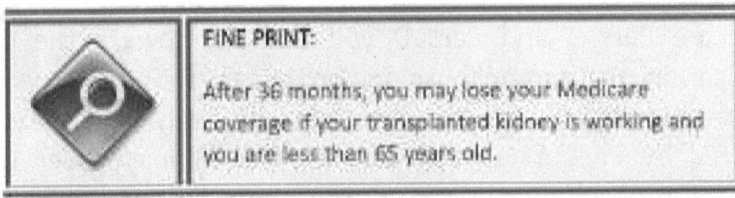

FINE PRINT:

After 36 months, you may lose your Medicare coverage if your transplanted kidney is working and you are less than 65 years old.

Part B coverage may even be used when you stay overnight in a hospital. This may seem confusing if you recall that Part A covers hospital expenses (another example of the fine print). Part A covers for inpatient care and Part B for outpatient care. Aren't you inpatient if you are IN the hospital? Not necessarily. We will save that discussion for Chapter 8.

Medicare Part D Medications

As stated earlier, the majority of your prescription medications are covered by Medicare Part D. Some Medicare Advantage plans also include Part D coverage.

At a minimum, Part D plans are required to cover at least two medications in each therapeutic drug class. For six of those classes — antidepressants, antipsychotics, chemotherapy agents, HIV/AIDS drugs, immunosuppressants, and seizure medications — nearly all medications will be covered.

Part D plans also cannot charge you more than 25 percent of the retail cost of any drug. If you need a more extensive plan or a plan that covers specifics medications, you may need to do some searching. It is possible that you could pay more than the basic premium which is $32.50 per month for 2019.

Simply put, Part D covers what Part B leaves behind. If someone had an organ transplant that was not covered by Medicare, their immunosuppressant drugs would be covered by Part D, not Part B. If someone wanted the Hepatitis B vaccine but was considered low risk, they would have to turn to their Part D coverage.

Medicare Part B and Part D will not pay toward the same medication. You can only use one or the other. This is especially important when it comes to certain hospital stays, i.e., those not covered by Part A (see Chapter 8). Part B may cover some medications administered in the hospital, usually those administered through an IV line. If you received Part D medications, however, be sure to make a copy of your bill and send them to your insurance plan. If the medications are on your formulary, your plan may reimburse you for them.

Negotiating Drug Costs

In addition to prescription medications, Medicare covers a percentage of the cost for other items used in the home, if it considers these items medically necessary (there's that magic phrase again).

Medical necessity is a key concept to understand and one that can set off more than a little debate. There is no all-inclusive list made available to the public, or to healthcare providers for that matter, that states what Medicare defines as medically necessary in every situation. If you come across such a list, please be sure to let me know—I want a copy

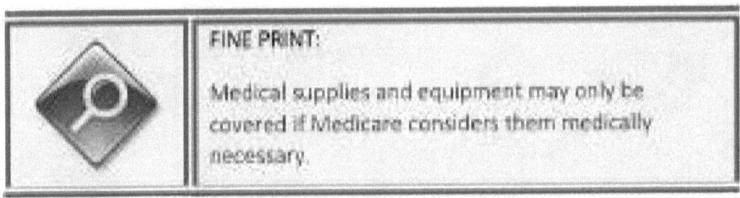

FINE PRINT:

Medical supplies and equipment may only be covered if Medicare considers them medically necessary.

Your healthcare provider needs to prescribe these items according to a specific diagnosis. Without a defined medical condition, the item will not be considered necessary in Medicare's eyes. The more specific the diagnosis, the more likely it will meet Medicare criteria, e.g., leg pain may not warrant use of crutches but a fracture of the left tibia may do it.

Medicare will often send forms to your doctor's office that requests information before they decide whether to cover your expenses. There is little room here for describing your personal circumstances. The questions are generally in yes/no or numerical format, e.g., a test result. If coverage is later denied based on the answers, a doctor may write an appeal letter on your behalf to see if they can convince Medicare that the prescription was medically necessary.

Part B covers the majority of outpatient utilities and requires a co-insurance be paid, usually at 20 percent cost.

According to the Centers for Disease Control and Prevention, in 2017, 30.3 million Americans had diabetes and 12.0 million of them were over the age of 65-years old. Part B covers many of the diabetic supplies needed to manage the condition. These may include insulin syringes and insulin needles. Glucometers to measure your sugar, control solutions to make sure the meter is working, lancets to prick your finger and tests strips to collect the blood sample are all included.

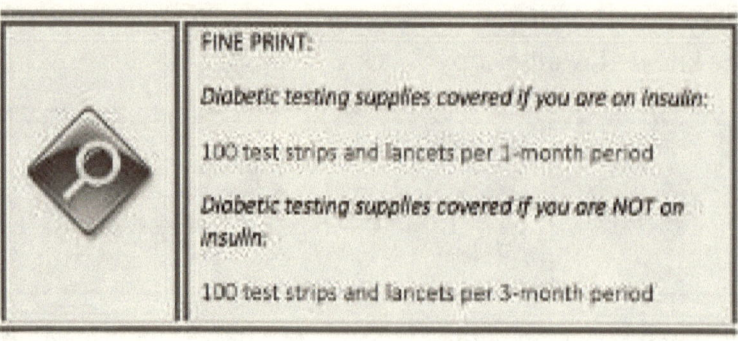

FINE PRINT:

Diabetic testing supplies covered if you are on insulin:

100 test strips and lancets per 1-month period

Diabetic testing supplies covered if you are NOT on insulin:

100 test strips and lancets per 3-month period

Do not take this to mean that you can check your blood sugar as much as you want. Based on the specific diagnosis your doctor provides (you would be stunned to know how many ICD-10 codes there are for diabetes), Medicare may set restrictions on how many supplies per month are covered. How well controlled your sugars are and whether or not you use insulin also comes into play.

If you are on insulin, you may be allowed 100 test strips and lancets per month. If you are not on insulin, that will extend to the same number of supplies over three months unless your doctor specifically documents a medical need.

Durable medical equipment is defined as equipment for the home that is intended for long-term use. There are a variety of supplies that may be covered under Part B.

Respiratory supplies may range from home oxygen to continuous positive airway pressure (CPAP) machines for sleep apnea. Nebulizer machines may also be covered.

Orthopedic supplies may include braces, shoe inserts, crutches, walkers and canes, though interestingly not white canes for the blind. A white cane designates a type of cane used by the visually impaired to help sense the environment around them. The white signifies to the public that the person using the cane is blind. Other covered items may include wheelchairs, both standard and motorized, and prosthetic devices.

For those with special needs, hospital beds, air mattresses, hydraulic lifts and bedside commodes may be indicated. Other supplies include infusion pumps, suction pumps, feeding pumps and ostomy supplies.

Please know that what is outlined in this chapter is not an exhaustive list of covered items.

Durable medical equipment, unfortunately, has been associated with increased cases of fraud. You may recall that there is no "limiting charge" applied to durable medical equipment and non-participating suppliers of that equipment. That means, they can charge far more than Medicare recommends. In 2016 alone, the U.S. health system spent $51.0 billion on durable medical equipment. It is estimated that 5 to 10 percent of those costs may be attributed to fraud.

It is no surprise that Medicare is taking steps to prevent improper payments. Starting in 2016, prior authorizations – a pre-approval process – have been put into effect on items considered at higher risk for being medically unnecessary or are more commonly associated with fraud. Many power wheelchairs and even joint prostheses are on that list. This process may delay the time it takes for you to access certain types of durable medical equipment.

Ambulance Transportation

Ambulance services may be covered if they are deemed medically necessary because other means of transportation would be considered unsafe or threatening to your health. For example, driving yourself to a hospital in the middle of a heart attack would pose a risk not only to you but to the public at large.

However, you cannot choose what hospital you go to by ambulance. You will be brought to the nearest available facility even if the hospital you usually use is only one minute further away in distance. You will pay the full cost of the ride if you request the other facility. Paramedic care may also be billed to the ambulance service.

FINE PRINT:

Ambulance services are covered, if medically necessary, to the nearest available facility (hospital or skilled nursing facility) which may or may not be the facility of your choice.

Ambulances are not deemed medically necessary to bring you to appointments, even if those appointments are for your health. The one exception is if you have end-stage renal disease, need dialysis, and require ambulance transportation to and from a dialysis facility. For this to be covered, however, your doctor needs to write an order that states it is medically necessary. Medicare will not cover the cost otherwise and the cost could be high.

Interestingly, Medicare Advantage plans may offer coverage for ride-sharing services like Lyft® and Uber® starting in 2019. This is based on a new CMS guideline that will allow Medicare Advantage plans to offer "supplemental benefits if they compensate for physical impairments, diminish the impact of injuries or health conditions, and/or reduce avoidable emergency room utilization." By providing transportation to and from physician appointments, Medicare Advantage plans are hoping they can keep beneficiaries healthy and decrease the need for hospital care. This will not be covered by Original Medicare.

It will save you money to do some research and find local resources that provide free transportation. You can call your healthcare provider, the American Red Cross or even your Town Hall to find information about services available where you live. In the worst scenario, it would even be better to call for a taxi cab than to foot an ambulance bill.

What's in a Visit?

You are offered a Welcome to Medicare Visit and it is FREE. You are offered an Annual Wellness Visit every year after that and it too is FREE. The Affordable Care Act has applauded itself time and again over adding this preventive medicine opportunity for its Medicare beneficiaries as well it should. These are wonderful offerings if you know how to use them to your benefit.

Before you giddily rub your hands together over the free sticker price, let me ask you a simple question. What does a visit mean to you?

One could think of a visit in a casual sense, a meeting where two people get together. This could be for a simple chat or talk. In medical terms, however, there are more implications. Meeting with a doctor implies an inspection or examination of some kind, although it would be nice to think that your doctor's bedside manner could also qualify as a chat or talk. The truth is these free visits offered to you by Medicare lean more to the talking variety than you may think.

Your expectation and the reality of what will happen at your visit may be skewed. Both of these visits, the Welcome to Medicare

Visit and the Annual Wellness Visit, do not include the doctor laying hands on you. There is no examination included.

Some people may find this surprising. After all, how can a medical visit intended to prevent disease not include a listen to your heart and lungs? How can a physician find cancer if he does not examine a woman's breast or a man's prostate?

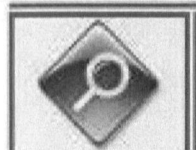

FINE PRINT:

The Welcome to Medicare visit and Annual Wellness visits do NOT include a physical examination.

While all these components may be important to early identification of disease, they are not the true intention behind these Medicare visits. Instead, these visits stand as a foundation from which to pursue the recommended screening interventions. Essentially, it is intended to be a consultation visit for discussion only.

This is where the nomenclature gets sticky. The word "visit" too often becomes interchanged with exam. Quite frankly, the office staff can sometimes be as confused as the patients scheduling appointments. In this case, though, the words do matter. It is not surprising when given the medical context. So when you sign up for your Welcome to Medicare "exam", know that you may be waiting for a long time—since it does not exist.

The Welcome to Medicare Visit

This visit is offered to you once and only once within the first year after signing up for Part B. This is the case whether or not you signed up at eligibility age. Covered under Part B, the visit itself is free but some of its individual components—in particular, screening tests that may be ordered at the visit—may not be.

First and foremost, your healthcare provider will sit down with you to discuss your history. To do a thorough job, this takes dedicated face time. Let us look to see what should be included.

Medical History – This should include a review of your medical problems, past and present, including surgeries. You are the only you. Understanding your personal health history to this point in your life will help guide your provider towards the most appropriate treatment and screening options.

Medication History – Understanding the purpose for each medication and how it interacts with your other medications is very important to minimize side effects. This includes not only prescription medications but over-the-counter medications as well. You would be surprised how many over-the-counter products, even certain vitamins, can interfere with your prescription drugs. To make the most of your visit, it is helpful for you to bring your medications in with you to your appointment.

Family History – You may be at higher risk for certain conditions based on your genes. Your healthcare provider should review your family history and specifically ask about medical conditions that tend to be inherited. This discussion will determine if you are at risk for certain diseases and again will guide treatment and screening options.

Social History – We are not talking about going to cocktail parties here, though that could be part of it. Your social history essentially addresses your lifestyle choices. Use of tobacco products, alcohol and drugs will be discussed. Your degree of physical activity will be taken into consideration. This is not an exhaustive list but stands as an opportunity for your healthcare provider to counsel you on lifestyle choices that could improve your health.

Vital signs are also an important part of any visit. Your healthcare provider or her nursing staff may be the one to take these measurements though this may be the only laying on of hands you get during the visit. This includes measuring your height, weight and blood pressure.

Your height and weight are used to calculate a number known as the body mass index (BMI) that categories your weight into underweight, normal weight, overweight or obese. Again, this is used as a tool to determine your health risk.

A simple vision screening test should also be performed at this visit. Do not confuse this to mean a full glaucoma screen. This screen may be as simple as reading an eye chart. Poor vision is a risk factor for falls and this is intended as a general safety assessment.

Your healthcare provider should also discuss your mental health and screen for depression. Depression is all too common and quality of life can be improved if the condition is identified early and addressed, either by counseling or medication if necessary.

It is not always easy to talk about advanced directives, i.e., end-of-life plans. The Welcome to Medicare Visit encourages you and your provider to discuss this in an open forum. It is not required that you make any final decisions at the visit but understanding your options is key to planning for your future.

Based on all this information gathering, your provider will now discuss with you what screening tests may be appropriate for you as an individual. You will be given a written list of tests that Medicare offers to you. Some of these screening tests may have costs attached. A detailed review of these preventive services will be discussed later in the chapter.

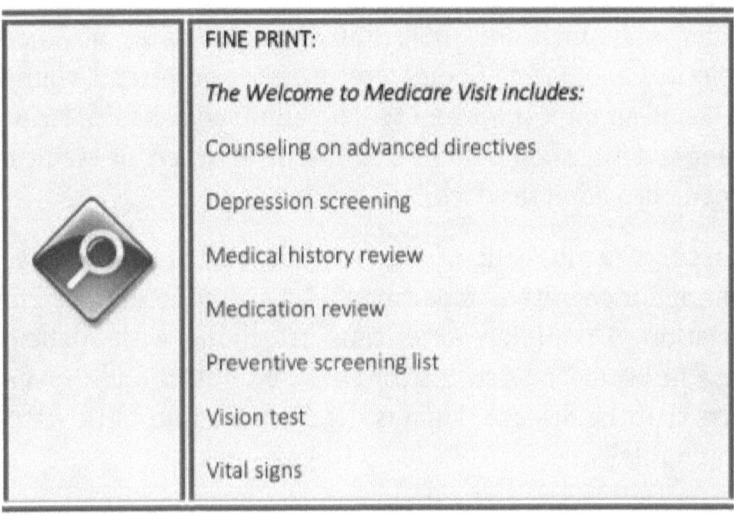

FINE PRINT:

The Welcome to Medicare Visit includes:

Counseling on advanced directives

Depression screening

Medical history review

Medication review

Preventive screening list

Vision test

Vital signs

The Annual Wellness Visit

Annual Wellness Visits are offered through Part B after you have been on Medicare for 12 months. This is not based on a calendar year but on an actual 12-month calendar. That is to say, having an Annual Wellness Visit one year in September and then the next in August is not covered. It is not required that you have had the Welcome to Medicare Visit to take advantage of these annual preventive visits.

This Annual Wellness Visit is essentially an extension of the Welcome to Medicare Visit as there is significant overlap between the two. Any changes to your personal history are reviewed. Vital signs are rechecked. Your preventive screening options are again outlined.

There are two features that make these visits distinct from the Welcome to Medicare Visit. The first of these is the health risk assessment or HRA. This is a questionnaire for you to complete that reviews topics ranging from your dietary habits to depression screening to safety in your home. Your healthcare provider may mail this questionnaire to you in advance for completion or you may complete it once you attend your visit. The HRA is an important tool to determine your health risks. It is also a mandatory component of the visit in order for Medicare to cover the provided services.

The second component of the Annual Wellness Visit involves screening for cognitive impairment. According to the Alzheimer's Association, 5.7 million Americans are living with Alzheimer's disease in 2018. The Centers for Disease Control and Prevention reports that the disease remains the sixth leading cause for death in our country.

Memory loss, confusion and dementia may be a result of Alzheimer's disease but many other conditions could be the cause. The truth is that the risk for cognitive impairment increases as we age and this affects how we respond to our environment. It becomes a matter of safety.

The Annual Wellness Visit offers your healthcare provider the opportunity to screen you for any changes to your cognitive status on a yearly basis. Medicare does not specify how your provider ought to complete the screening, only that screening is indicated. There are many approaches a provider may take to complete the screening. That said, do not be too surprised if you are asked to spell words backwards, to subtract numbers, or to draw a clock.

The one aspect of your Welcome to Medicare Visit that is not continued in your Annual Wellness Visits is a vision test. This is unfortunate since vision tends to get worse as you get older.

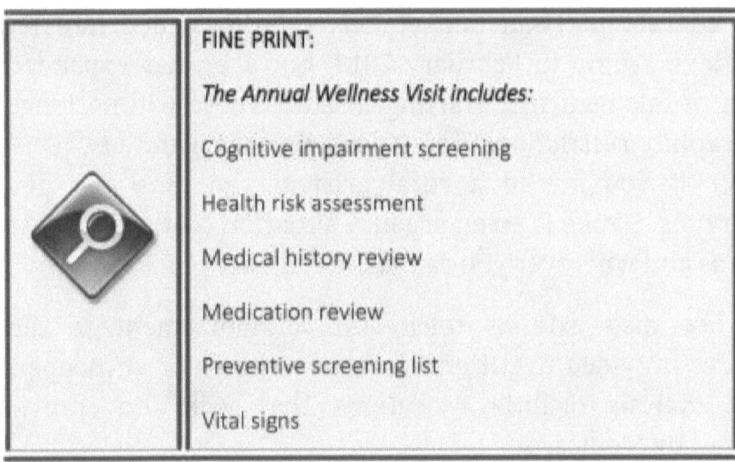

FINE PRINT:

The Annual Wellness Visit includes:

Cognitive impairment screening

Health risk assessment

Medical history review

Medication review

Preventive screening list

Vital signs

One would think vision tests should be covered annually for safety reasons. Your healthcare provider may offer you a vision test at your Annual Wellness Visit but be aware that it may not be free of charge.

Telemedicine Visits

Telemedicine, also referred to as telehealth, is becoming more popular. This type of visit allows you to see a healthcare provider without actually being at the same physical location. Instead, you communicate using real-time audio and video.

Traditionally, Medicare covered the service with restrictions. If you lived in a rural area, you would be covered for a telemedicine visit at a 20 percent Part B co-insurance if it took place at a doctor's office, a hospital, a critical access hospital (CAH), a rural health clinic, a federally qualified health center, a hospital-based or critical access hospital-based dialysis facility, a skilled nursing facility, or a community mental health center. That's right, you cannot take advantage of this service from the comfort of your own home.

The federal Bipartisan Budget Act of 2018, signed into law by President Trump in February 2018, however, has expanded the reach of telemedicine. Starting in 2019, there will no longer be geographic restrictions for telestroke services, i.e., it won't matter if you are in a rural area at the time you develop symptoms. Stroke is an emergency situation that requires care as soon as and wherever you can get it.

The law also extends telehealth reimbursement to dialysis services provided to patients located at home or at independent renal dialysis facilities, locations that were not previously covered by Medicare.

Finally, Medicare Advantage plans will be able to add telehealth services as a basic benefit starting in 2020.

Physical, Occupational and Speech Therapy

Physical Therapy (PT), Speech-Language Pathology services (SLP) and Occupational Therapy (OT) are services frequently required for those who suffer from orthopedic problems, rheumatologic problems, strokes and other disabling conditions. Part B covers these outpatient services with a 20 percent co-insurance (you pay 20 percent of the visit cost).

Medicare used to have a Therapy Cap Limit. After the monetary cap was reached, you would be responsible for paying the full cost of therapy out of pocket. Thankfully, this cap was removed in 2018.

Now Medicare only requires that your therapist confirm that your care is medically necessary once a certain amount of money has been spent each year, $2,010 for Physical Therapy and Speech-Language Pathology services combined and for $2,010 for Occupational Therapy in 2018. This amount includes the 20 percent you spend for your visits as well as the 80 percent Medicare pays.

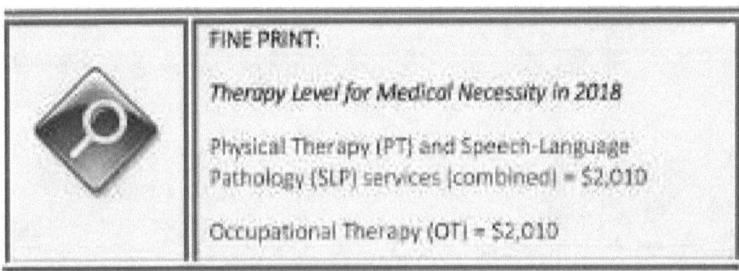

FINE PRINT:

Therapy Level for Medical Necessity in 2018

Physical Therapy (PT) and Speech-Language Pathology (SLP) services (combined) = $2,010

Occupational Therapy (OT) = $2,010

To get a sense of these costs, Healthcare Bluebook estimates the charge for an initial Physical Therapy visit to be $118 and follow-up visits at $80. Of course, this will vary based on what services are actually provided at those sessions and where you live in the country. Some therapists use different techniques and equipment such as ultrasound, massage and traction that may add extra fees for any given visit.

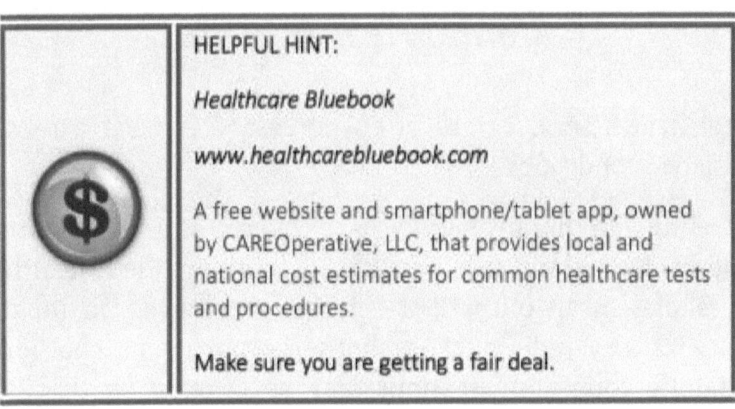

HELPFUL HINT:

Healthcare Bluebook

www.healthcarebluebook.com

A free website and smartphone/tablet app, owned by CAREOperative, LLC, that provides local and national cost estimates for common healthcare tests and procedures.

Make sure you are getting a fair deal.

Because of this variability, I would look to these Healthcare Bluebook estimates more as a minimum baseline cost in this scenario. It may be a more reliable guide for other healthcare costs such as laboratory tests, imaging studies and surgical procedures in your local area.

Defining medically necessity lies in the hands of the therapist providing your services. They must carefully state the reasons their services are appropriate and necessary for your recovery and clearly document this in your medical chart for each visit. Otherwise, Medicare will not pay to continue those services.

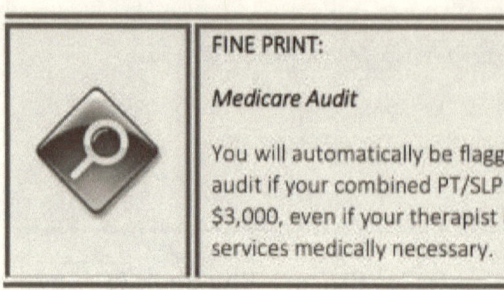

FINE PRINT:

Medicare Audit

You will automatically be flagged for a Medicare audit if your combined PT/SLP or OT costs exceed $3,000, even if your therapist has deemed the services medically necessary.

However, know that your chart will be flagged for an automatic Medicare audit if your services exceed $3,000 for combined Physical Therapy and Speech-Language Pathology services or for Occupational Therapy services.

Mental Health Visits

Mental health services are often necessary to treat a range of psychiatric conditions.

Counseling and therapy services are covered at a co-insurance of 20 percent if they are provided by a qualified healthcare professional in an outpatient setting (not during an inpatient hospitalization). Individual psychotherapy, group psychotherapy, and family counseling sessions may be covered by the Part B benefit.

Qualified professionals include physicians, physician assistants, nurse practitioners, certified nurse-midwives, clinical nurse specialists, clinical psychologists or clinical social workers.

If you require mental health care while you are hospitalized as an inpatient (see Chapter 8), Part A will pay for those services. However, there is a lifetime cap on how many days Part A will cover. In that case, let's hope you will not require more than 190 days of inpatient psychiatric hospital care.

Advance Beneficiary Notice of Non-Coverage

(ABN)

It is important that you discuss the costs for any tests or procedures performed with your healthcare provider. This is especially true for Physical Therapy, Speech-Language Pathology Services and Occupational Therapy since there is a risk that Medicare may not consider them medically necessary. In fact, your provider has an obligation to tell you if there is a risk that Medicare will not cover the costs of any tests, procedures or services that are being ordered.

This information should be provided to you in written form as an Advance Beneficiary Notice (ABN) of Non-Coverage and given to you BEFORE any test or procedure is completed. The same goes for ambulance transportation. You will be required to sign this form as acknowledgement that Medicare may not pay for the service. It essentially becomes a contract stating that you agree to pay any charges not covered by Medicare.

If you choose not to sign the ABN, the healthcare provider reserves the right not to proceed with services. For obvious reasons, he wants to get paid. If he forgets to have you sign one, he is out of luck.

If an ABN is not given to you in advance of the tests and procedures provided and Medicare does not pay for the services, you are NOT financially liable for the cost of the studies.

I will add a caveat here. Some healthcare providers may have you sign an informed consent form for a procedure instead of an official ABN. It may make mention of possible non-coverage of the test within that form. If you sign it, you may be responsible for the costs, even if there is not a formal ABN. Always read any document before you sign and ask questions if there is anything on it you don't understand.

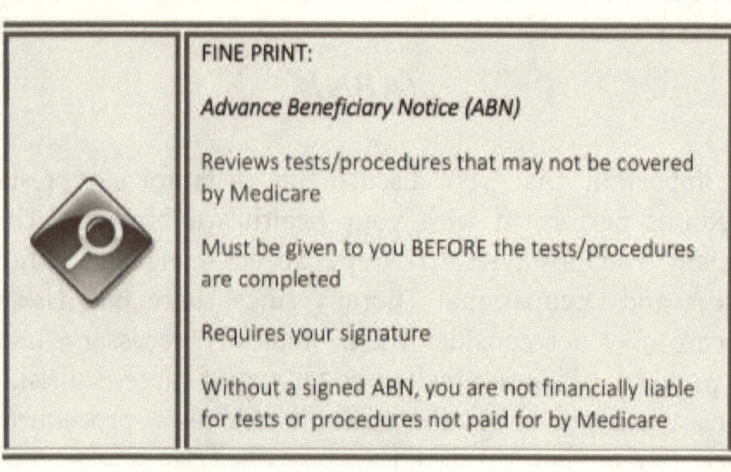

FINE PRINT:

Advance Beneficiary Notice (ABN)

Reviews tests/procedures that may not be covered by Medicare

Must be given to you BEFORE the tests/procedures are completed

Requires your signature

Without a signed ABN, you are not financially liable for tests or procedures not paid for by Medicare

There is a distinction to be made between the healthcare provider ordering a test and the one actually performing the test. Your provider may order a test but if he does not perform it in his office, he is not the one required to offer you an ABN. The provider or facility that completes the service is the one responsible. Simply stated, your healthcare provider is responsible for what he does, not for what others do.

The most common example of this occurs with blood work. Your healthcare provider may send you to a laboratory facility to have tests drawn. The laboratory facility is obligated to provide you with an ABN because they are the one taking the risk that they will not be paid for their services. Likewise, when a provider refers you to a specialist for care, the specialist becomes responsible for any tests or procedures he performs.

In the case of a colonoscopy, the provider performing the study must offer you an ABN or an informed consent form that outlines the same. This becomes especially important when it comes to screening colonoscopies. As you will learn in the following chapter, a screening colonoscopy may be converted to a diagnostic one if an abnormality is found during the procedure. The difference is that the screening colonoscopy is outright free to you and the diagnostic colonoscopy requires you to pay a Medicare co-insurance of 20 percent. That could be hundreds of dollars depending on where in the country you have the procedure performed.

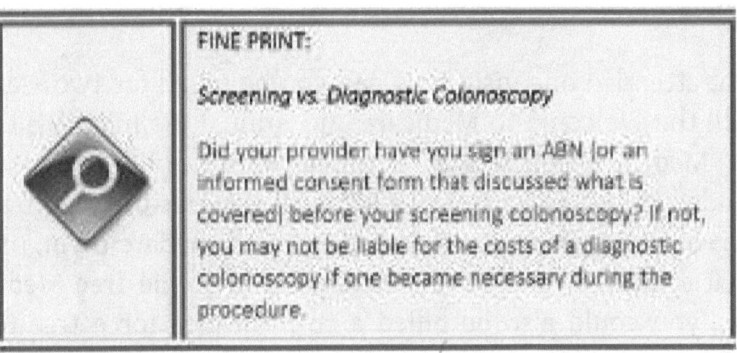

FINE PRINT:

Screening vs. Diagnostic Colonoscopy

Did your provider have you sign an ABN (or an informed consent form that discussed what is covered) before your screening colonoscopy? If not, you may not be liable for the costs of a diagnostic colonoscopy if one became necessary during the procedure.

If the person performing the study does not provide you with an ABN to discuss the possibility for a diagnostic colonoscopy BEFORE the procedure is completed, you will not be liable for those extra costs.

Medicare Audits

It frequently happens that a person will ask their healthcare provider to perform additional services at their Welcome to Medicare Visit or their Annual Wellness Visit. After all, it saves him time from having to come to the office for another visit. The healthcare provider may agree to do this, if time allows, but this person must be aware that he may be charged the cost of an extra visit.

If you attended one visit, how can you be billed for two? As you recall, the Welcome to Medicare and Annual Wellness Visits are free. Medicare specifically outlines what services are to be provided at these visits. Any additional services are not covered and require another visit be billed to accommodate them. In this scenario, even if you have scheduled one of the free Medicare visits, you could also be billed a co-insurance for a traditional office visit. The intent is to avoid Medicare fraud and fines.

Medicare reserves the right to randomly audit charts in a medical office. The purpose for this is to reduce fraud. As sad as it is, there have been excessive abuses to the system in the past and Medicare has recovered billions of dollars by ramping up audits and investigations.

When billing errors are noted in a chart, Medicare fines the provider for the infringement but on a larger scale, a percentage scale. For example, if Medicare audited 10 charts and found 1 chart with errors, they assume that 1 out of every 10 charts had a billing error. Medicare will then fine the provider based on 10 percent of his total Medicare practice. If the average patient panel is 2,000 patients, that can lead to excessive fines. One error can lead to a heavy financial burden for a medical office.

The Medicare Fraud Strike Force was established in 2007 and for good reason. Far too many people are abusing the system, taking hard earned dollars away from Medicare. In 2017 alone, the federal government recovered $2.6 billion from fraudulent transactions.

While allowing you to have a follow-up visit at the same time as a Wellness visit may not seem to be a dastardly deed, Medicare still does not want to give away something for nothing. You pay nothing for the Welcome and Wellness visits but Medicare is paying your provider on the back end. That is to say, your provider bills Medicare for services rendered.

After an audit, Medicare may not acknowledge the visit you received as one of the covered Welcome or Wellness visits and may penalize that healthcare provider or its office for billing as such. Medicare may do this by denying your provider payment for the visit, subjecting the office to fines or otherwise.

How Medicare chooses to address these issues is, and may always be, a work-in-progress but trust me, your provider does not want to get on Medicare's bad side. It puts his entire medical practice at risk.

It can be all too easy to demand more from your healthcare provider but you must understand that they have as much to gain or lose as you do when it comes to Medicare's evolving processes. It is more important that you establish a healthy physician-patient relationship and discuss with them any concerns you have. Your provider should equally be open about what he can and cannot do. Together, hopefully you can learn what works best for both of you.

Preventive Services for Cardiovascular

Disease

Cardiovascular disease is more than prevalent in our society. It includes diseases such as coronary artery disease, congestive heart failure, angina, hypertension, aortic aneurysm and stroke among other conditions. According to the Center for Disease Control (CDC), there are 610,000 deaths from heart disease each year. Each year approximately 525,000 have their first heart attack, and 210,000 people who have had one in the past have another one.

Doing what we can to minimize these diseases plays a major role in keeping you healthy and may reduce healthcare costs for the future, for both you and the healthcare system at large.

Medicare appreciates the importance of screening for risk factors that could lead to cardiovascular disease. For one, blood pressure screening is performed at every Annual Wellness Visit free of charge. Based on these results, your healthcare provider may counsel you with diet and lifestyle recommendations to reduce your blood pressure. This becomes an opportunity to discuss whether medication options are appropriate for your situation.

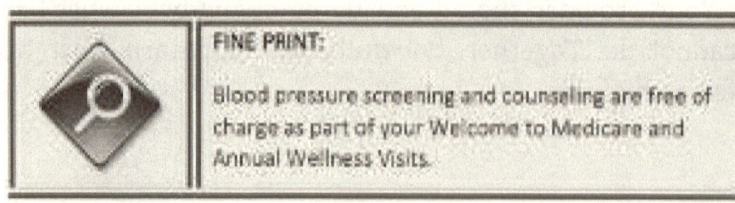

FINE PRINT:

Blood pressure screening and counseling are free of charge as part of your Welcome to Medicare and Annual Wellness Visits.

The amount of fat in our bodies can contribute to blockage of arteries, possibly leading to heart attack and stroke. Part B coverage allows for screening of cholesterol, lipids and triglycerides once every five years. This test is best performed when you are fasting, if possible.

Medicare does not take into consideration whether or not you already have known cholesterol or lipid problems. Part B covers the screening test free of charge only once every five years. Any additional lipid screenings required in between those time periods will be charged to Part B as a non-preventive service.

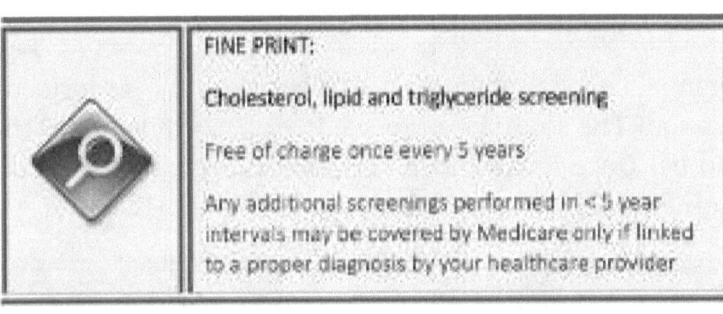

FINE PRINT:

Cholesterol, lipid and triglyceride screening

Free of charge once every 5 years

Any additional screenings performed in < 5 year intervals may be covered by Medicare only if linked to a proper diagnosis by your healthcare provider

Depending on what diagnosis your healthcare provider links to those additional tests, Medicare may or may not cover the cost of the test. Examples of covered diagnoses include coronary atherosclerosis, diabetes, essential hypertension, heart failure, hypertriglyceridemia, mixed hyperlipidemia, pure hypercholesterolemia, obesity and transient cerebral ischemia.

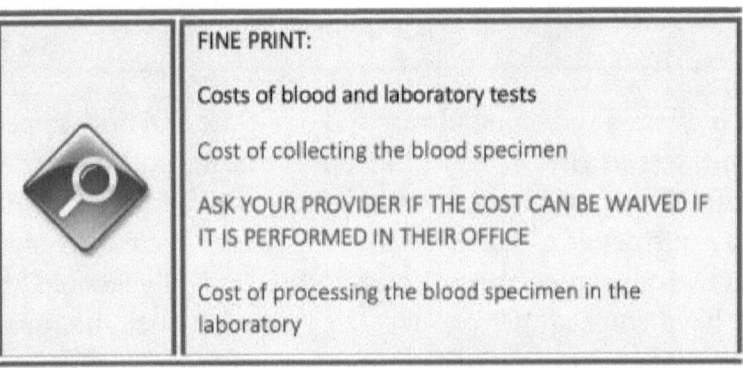

FINE PRINT:

Costs of blood and laboratory tests

Cost of collecting the blood specimen

ASK YOUR PROVIDER IF THE COST CAN BE WAIVED IF IT IS PERFORMED IN THEIR OFFICE

Cost of processing the blood specimen in the laboratory

It is important to understand the added costs of blood tests. First, there is the cost of collecting the blood from your veins – the needles, the test tubes, the skilled personnel to gather the sample. Second, there is the actual cost of processing the blood sample in the laboratory. Part B may offer coverage for the latter and not the former, though Medicare may cover this cost if it is for a test considered medically necessary.

If the blood draw is done in your healthcare provider's office, it may be possible for the office to waive the draw fee. Your provider does not have the authority to ask an outside laboratory facility to waive this fee.

Abdominal aortic aneurysm screening is performed by ultrasound. The study looks to see if your aorta is larger than it should be. Once it reaches a certain size, it may be at risk for rupturing, which could be fatal.

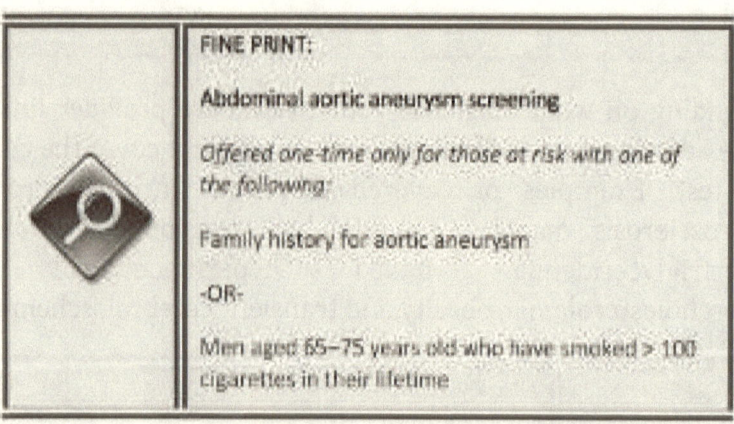

FINE PRINT:

Abdominal aortic aneurysm screening

Offered one-time only for those at risk with one of the following:

Family history for aortic aneurysm

-OR-

Men aged 65–75 years old who have smoked > 100 cigarettes in their lifetime

Part B offers a screening ultrasound one-time and only to people it considers at risk. The risk factors Medicare outlines are very specific. The first of these considerations is based on a known family history for aortic aneurysms. The second is gender specific. For men between the ages of 65 and 75 years old, those who have smoked 100 or more cigarettes in their lifetime are considered at risk.

Preventive Services for Diabetes

According to the American Diabetes Association, 30.3 million Americans had diabetes in 2015. When looking at different age categories it was found 25.2 percent of people 65 years of age and older had the condition. Diabetes cost the United States $327 billion in direct medical costs and reduced productivity in 2017.

Complications of diabetes are varied but all too common. The high sugars associated with diabetes can attach to small- and large-sized blood vessels. This can lead to lead to heart and kidney disease. Your vision may be impaired when sugars collect on the retina. Nerve damage or neuropathy can develop causing pain or numbness.

Part B allows for screening of diabetes twice per year if certain conditions are met. High blood pressure, high cholesterol, high triglycerides, high sugar levels and obesity, defined as a BMI > 30, may be associated with a diagnosis of diabetes.

Other risk factors for diabetes include age greater than 65 years old, being overweight (BMI 25–30), or having gestational diabetes. Diabetes in pregnancy is frequently associated with diabetes later in life. Mothers with infants born at weights greater than 9 lbs. may have had glucose problems during their pregnancy, even if they passed their gestational diabetes screening. A family history for diabetes may contribute to risk for developing diabetes as well.

Medicare does not specify how to screen for diabetes. Screening may be done with a simple fasting glucose blood test: levels greater than 126 on two separate tests diagnose diabetes. Non-fasting glucose levels may be suggestive for the disorder if they are greater than 200. Some healthcare providers may use a blood test called the hemoglobin A1C. Levels greater than 6.5 on two separate tests are indicative of diabetes. An oral glucose tolerance test measures your body's response to sugar by measuring your blood sugar before and after ingesting a fixed amount of glucose; this test is labor intensive and most commonly done in pregnant women.

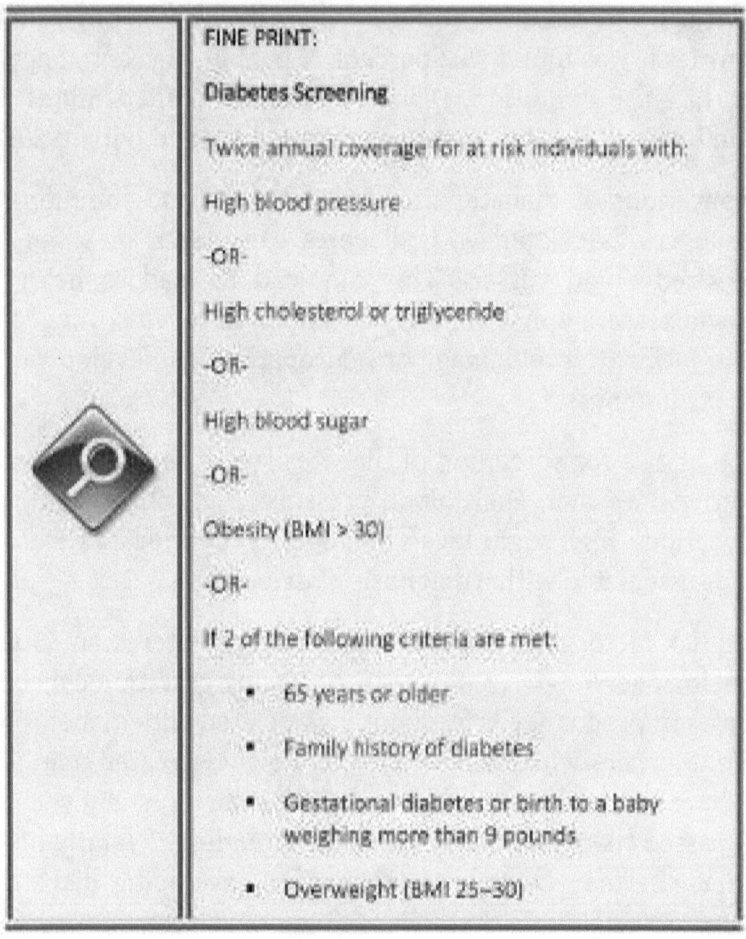

FINE PRINT:

Diabetes Screening

Twice annual coverage for at risk individuals with:

High blood pressure

-OR-

High cholesterol or triglyceride

-OR-

High blood sugar

-OR-

Obesity (BMI > 30)

-OR-

If 2 of the following criteria are met:

- 65 years or older
- Family history of diabetes
- Gestational diabetes or birth to a baby weighing more than 9 pounds
- Overweight (BMI 25–30)

For those confirmed to have diabetes, it is important to understand how to best manage the disease to minimize complications. Part B covers diabetic self-management training to educate diabetic patients about the disease. This training may include information about a diabetic diet, how to check blood sugar levels and for those requiring insulin, how to appropriately inject insulin.

Part B covers up to 10 hours of initial training if sessions are ordered by a healthcare provider. In subsequent years, Part B will cover up to two extra hours per year in group sessions of 2–20 people for sessions lasting 30 minutes or more. If group sessions are not locally available or if a provider indicates a medical reason why group sessions would not be appropriate, for example psychiatric reasons, an exception can be made to the requirement. Each visit requires a co-insurance payment of 20 percent.

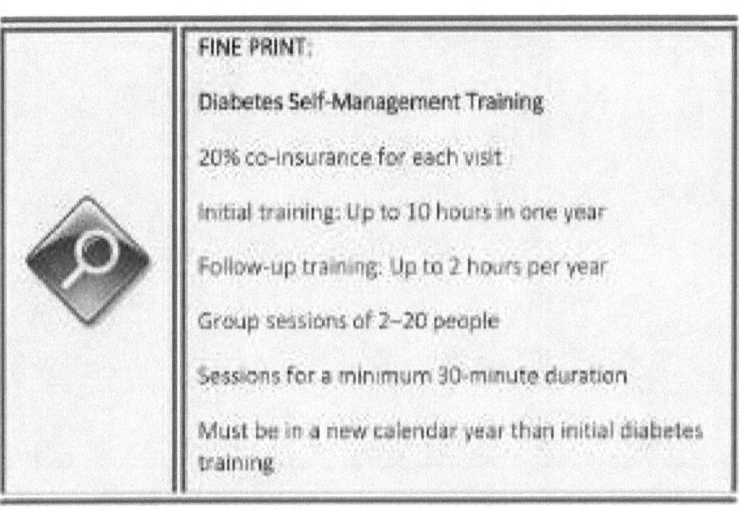

FINE PRINT:

Diabetes Self-Management Training

20% co-insurance for each visit

Initial training: Up to 10 hours in one year

Follow-up training: Up to 2 hours per year

Group sessions of 2–20 people

Sessions for a minimum 30-minute duration

Must be in a new calendar year than initial diabetes training

Preventive Services for Infection

Infectious diseases are essential part of preventive medicine. The spreading of disease becomes a public health issue. Medicare has targeted specific infections for coverage.

The United States Preventive Services Task Force (USPSTF) announced its recommendation in June 2013 to screen for hepatitis C in people at high risk for the disease or for people born between 1945 and 1965. In March 2014, Medicare agreed to include this screening in its preventive services.

People at high risk include those who have ever used injected illicit drugs or who received a blood transfusion before 1992. Annual screening is covered for those who continue to use illicit drugs. For those not considered at high risk but who were born between 1945 and 1965, screening is offered one time only. An epidemiologic study found a higher prevalence of hepatitis C in this age group.

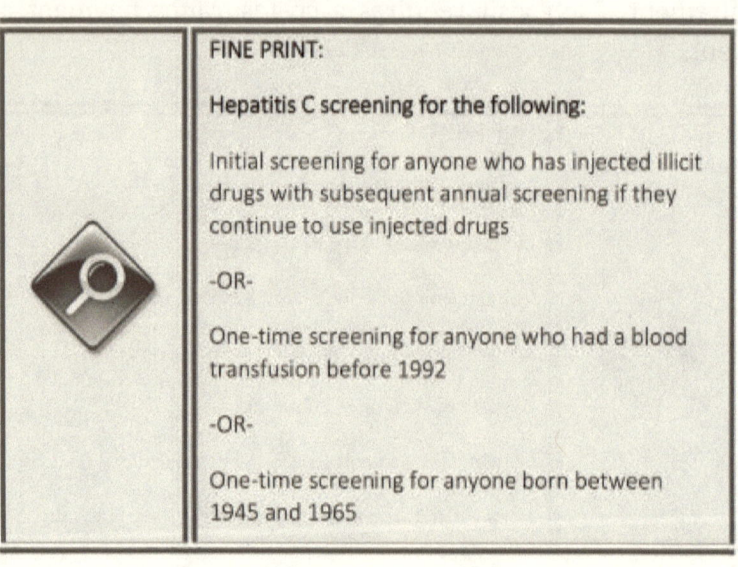

FINE PRINT:

Hepatitis C screening for the following:

Initial screening for anyone who has injected illicit drugs with subsequent annual screening if they continue to use injected drugs

-OR-

One-time screening for anyone who had a blood transfusion before 1992

-OR-

One-time screening for anyone born between 1945 and 1965

Sexually transmitted infections (STI) include chlamydia, gonorrhea and syphilis. Hepatitis B may be an STI although it can also be transmitted in other ways. Other STIs are not specified by Medicare and may not be covered. These may include herpes and mycoplasma infections among other infections. Part B covers screening of the specified STIs once annually for sexually active Medicare beneficiaries who are considered at risk. Risk factors are not clearly defined by Medicare but may include unprotected sexual intercourse with multiple partners and partner infidelity.

Taken one step further, those at risk may continue to be at risk if steps are not taken to change their behaviors. Medicare Part B covers behavioral counseling sessions to address these issues. Up to two separate face-to-face visits may be covered for up to 30 minutes per session. This counseling is covered in the outpatient setting but is not covered as a preventive service if the counseling is performed in the hospital or in a skilled nursing facility. In those settings, charges will apply.

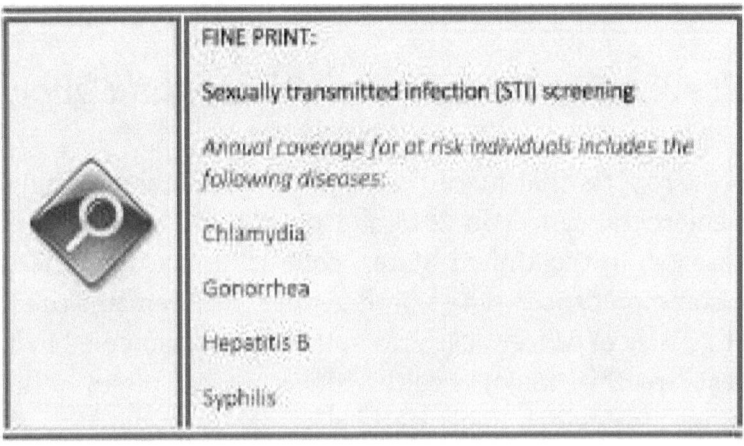

FINE PRINT:

Sexually transmitted infection (STI) screening

Annual coverage for at risk individuals includes the following diseases:

Chlamydia

Gonorrhea

Hepatitis B

Syphilis

Human immunodeficiency virus or HIV may be more common than you think. In 2015, the Centers for Disease Control and Prevention reported that 1.2 million Americans were infected with HIV and as many as 15 percent of them were unaware they even had the virus. Medicare Part B covers HIV screening once annually for any Medicare beneficiary at risk and for any who simply request the test.

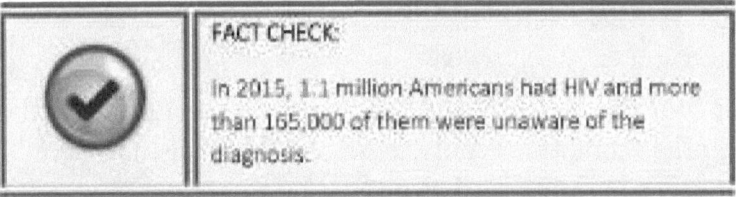

FACT CHECK:

In 2015, 1.1 million Americans had HIV and more than 165,000 of them were unaware of the diagnosis.

Pregnancy is considered a special scenario. After all, the mother's health is not only at risk but also that of the baby. Medicare Part B covers STI and HIV screening over the course of the pregnancy.

Though much controversy has sprung up over vaccinations in recent years, vaccinations have been proven to save lives and decrease the spread of infection. Medicare covers flu shots, pneumonia shots and hepatitis B shots for appropriate candidates. The details of this are discussed in Chapter 4 under "Medicare Part B Medications".

Preventive Services for Colorectal Cancer

The CDC reports that more than 140,788 people were diagnosed with colorectal cancer in 2015 and more than 52,396 died from the disease. In the United States, colorectal cancer is the third most common cancer across both genders and remains the third leading cause of cancer death for both men and women. Medicare appreciates this major health concern and offers different screening strategies to look for the disease.

Screening opportunities begin at age 50 for both men and women. Each test has different risks associated with it. Your healthcare provider will guide you towards the best option for screening depending on your medical history.

A simple rectal examination performed in the office can be used to check for blood in the stool. Alternatively, your provider may supply you with "stool cards" to collect samples of your stool at home and bring back to the office for analysis.

This screening is known as a fecal occult blood test. A positive result could be indicative of underlying colorectal cancer though many other conditions could cause blood in the stool as well. This is the least invasive testing and can be checked once annually free of charge. If it is positive, your healthcare provider will likely recommend additional screening with another test. Be aware that there can be false-positive results based on what you eat. Red meat, cantaloupe, radishes, and turnips are notorious for this so it may be best to refrain from ingesting these foods in the days preceding your test. Please note that a negative screening test does not exclude a diagnosis of colorectal cancer.

As of 2015, Medicare covers DNA testing of the stool every 3 years for people at low risk for colon cancer. Symptoms such as blood in the stool or gastrointestinal complaints, such as abdominal pain, will exclude you from this type of screening. Medical conditions such as colon polyps, Crohn's disease, ulcerative colitis or a family history for colon polyps/cancer can also exclude coverage of the test.

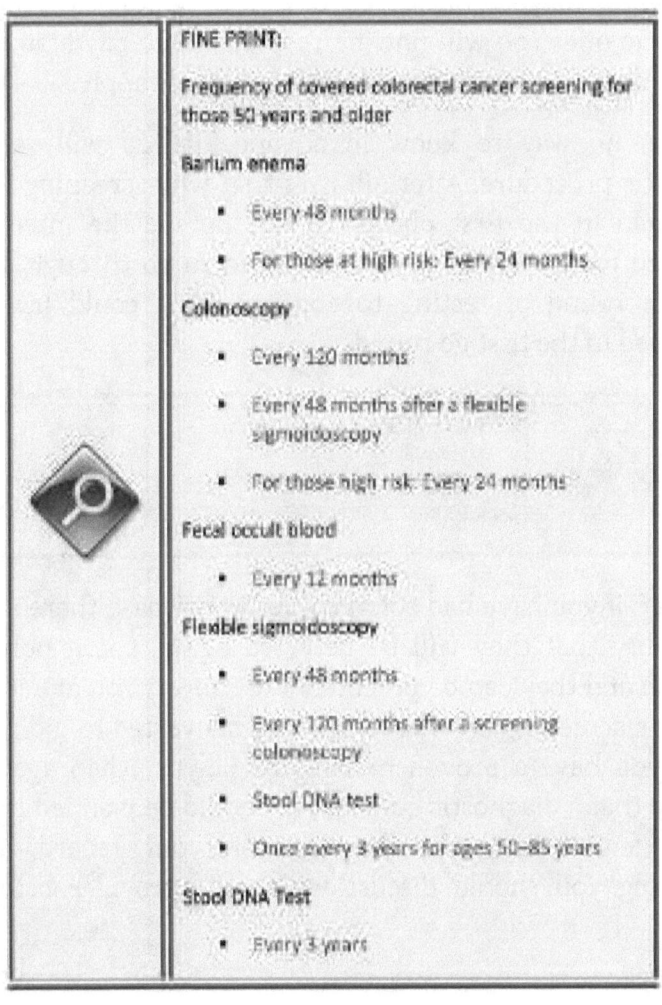

FINE PRINT:

Frequency of covered colorectal cancer screening for those 50 years and older

Barium enema

- Every 48 months
- For those at high risk: Every 24 months

Colonoscopy

- Every 120 months
- Every 48 months after a flexible sigmoidoscopy
- For those high risk: Every 24 months

Fecal occult blood

- Every 12 months

Flexible sigmoidoscopy

- Every 48 months
- Every 120 months after a screening colonoscopy
- Stool DNA test
- Once every 3 years for ages 50–85 years

Stool DNA Test

- Every 3 years

Flexible sigmoidoscopy and colonoscopy are more invasive but provide the most information. A camera is inserted into the rectum and used to directly visualize the colon. Sigmoidoscopy extends only to the lower part of the colon whereas colonoscopy extends further into the colon. When used for screening purposes, these tests are free under Medicare Part B.

However, do not be surprised if you end up with a bill just the same. In the case that a suspicious area is detected during the examination and intervention is pursued, such as a biopsy, the study is no longer considered a screening test—it becomes a diagnostic one. You will now be responsible to pay a 20 percent co-insurance. However, the deductible will not apply.

There is no way to know in advance if you will require a diagnostic procedure. After all, isn't that why screening is being performed in the first place? To not pursue the intervention would be foolhardy, as you would need to go through another vigorous round of testing to confirm what could have been completed in the first go round.

FINE PRINT:

Your screening colonoscopy could be converted to a diagnostic colonoscopy during the procedure.

However, if you have had colon polyps in the past, there is a high probability that they will be detected again. Colon polyps are common and they can be precursors to cancer. You are at higher risk for a screening colonoscopy being converted to a diagnostic one if you have a proven history for polyps. Then again, it is possible that a diagnostic colonoscopy could be planned from the get-go if you have the diagnosis on your record. This is something you should discuss with your provider before the study.

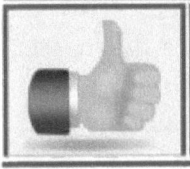

The frequency of screening will vary based on which test is pursued. For those at normal risk, flexible sigmoidoscopies and colonoscopies may be performed every 48 months or 120 months, respectively. If a colonoscopy was performed previously, it could be followed up by a flexible sigmoidoscopy in 120 months. If a flexible sigmoidoscopy was performed previously, it could be followed up by a colonoscopy in 48 months. For those at higher risk for colorectal cancer, colonoscopies may be pursued every 24 months.

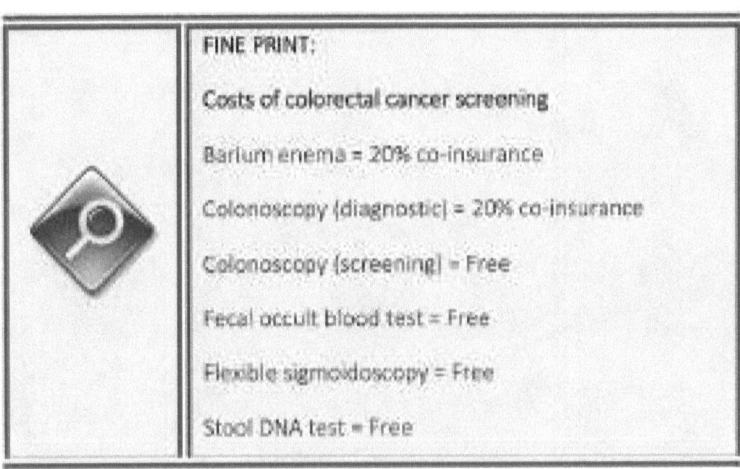

FINE PRINT:

Costs of colorectal cancer screening

Barium enema = 20% co-insurance

Colonoscopy (diagnostic) = 20% co-insurance

Colonoscopy (screening) = Free

Fecal occult blood test = Free

Flexible sigmoidoscopy = Free

Stool DNA test = Free

Remember that your doctor must accept assignment for these screening tests to be free of charge. Otherwise, you will be charged a Part B co-insurance.

If your risk for complications is considered too high for either procedure based on your medical history, your provider may recommend an alternative test called a barium enema. A barium enema inserts dye into the rectum via an enema and looks for irregular shapes or narrowing on x-ray that could be suggestive for colon cancer. Like the fecal occult test, positive results may be suggestive for colorectal cancer but may not be diagnostic. You and your doctor can decide whether or not to pursue more invasive testing if your results are abnormal.

Preventive Services for Women

With the advent of Pap smear screening, cervical cancer rates have considerably declined over the years. The CDC reports that 12,845 women were diagnosed with cervical cancer in 2015 while more than 4,175 women died from the disease in the same year.

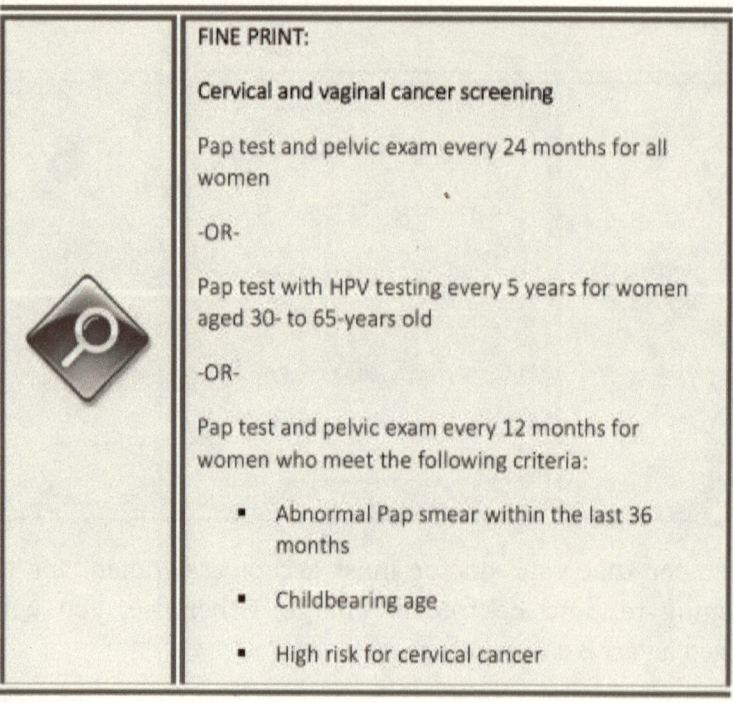

FINE PRINT:

Cervical and vaginal cancer screening

Pap test and pelvic exam every 24 months for all women

-OR-

Pap test with HPV testing every 5 years for women aged 30- to 65-years old

-OR-

Pap test and pelvic exam every 12 months for women who meet the following criteria:

- Abnormal Pap smear within the last 36 months

- Childbearing age

- High risk for cervical cancer

Part B covers cervical cancer screening with a Pap smear test every 24 months for all women and every 12 months for women if they meet high risk criteria. These high risk criteria may include a woman being of childbearing age or having an abnormal Pap smear test result within the last 36 months. In 2016, Medicare added an additional screening option. Women aged 30 to 65 years old can get a Pap smear with human papilloma virus (HPV) testing once every five years instead of the standard Pap smear every 24 months. HPV is a virus that has been shown to cause to cervical cancer.

Pap smear screening is not indicated for women who have had their cervix removed by way of a hysterectomy so long as the hysterectomy was not performed because of cancer.

Pelvic exams enable the healthcare provider to assess the vulva, the vagina, the uterus and the ovaries. Medicare recommends the exam every 24 months to screen for vaginal cancer in all women and annually if a woman is considered to be at risk, as for cervical cancer screening.

Interestingly, in 2016, the U.S. Preventive Services Task Force (USPSTF) stated there was insufficient evidence to support the use of pelvic exams for screening in women who did not have symptoms. Medicare, at the time of this publication, had not changed their coverage policy for pelvic exams.

Breast cancer is the most common non-skin cancer in women according to the CDC and the second leading cause of cancer death for the gender. In 2015, approximately 242,476 women were diagnosed with breast cancer while approximately 41,523 women died from the disease. Clinical breast exams are covered every 24 months (2 years) under Medicare Part B. Mammograms, however, have become the standard for identification of early breast cancer.

A woman becomes eligible for one baseline mammogram screening between the ages of 35 and 39 years old. At 40 years old, she becomes eligible for routine screening every year. Medicare covers the cost of screening mammograms but a co-insurance of 20 percent is required for diagnostic mammograms. The Part B deductible also applies in this case.

The imaging modalities are different in that diagnostic mammograms may have better resolution to look at a suspicious area of tissue. A diagnostic mammogram may be indicated if looking at a suspicious breast mass or for following someone who has had a history for breast cancer. Medicare does not cover ultrasounds or MRIs as preventive screening options for breast cancer.

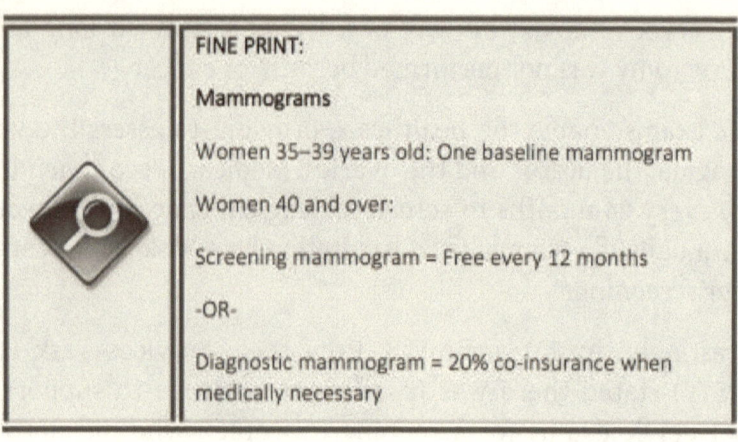

FINE PRINT:

Mammograms

Women 35–39 years old: One baseline mammogram

Women 40 and over:

Screening mammogram = Free every 12 months

-OR-

Diagnostic mammogram = 20% co-insurance when medically necessary

Similar to screening and diagnostic colonoscopies, how your provider orders the test will determine how much you pay. You have the right to know. Be proactive and ask how the study is being ordered.

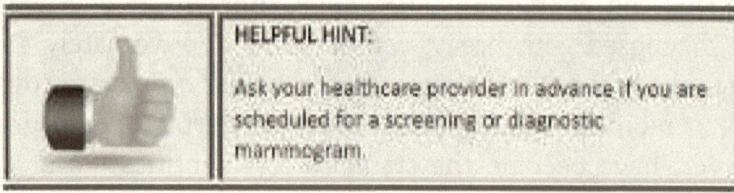

HELPFUL HINT:

Ask your healthcare provider in advance if you are scheduled for a screening or diagnostic mammogram.

Preventive Services for Men

Prostate cancer is the most common non-skin cancer in men according to the CDC. In 2015, 183,529 men were diagnosed with prostate cancer while 28,848 men died from the disease. Screening for prostate cancer has become more controversial in recent years. Debates have been waged on whether early detection of prostate cancer actually saves lives.

Prostate specific antigen (PSA) is a simple blood test that measures a protein that is secreted by the prostate. While elevations in PSA can be an indicator for prostate cancer, it can also be caused by infections and other problems relating to the prostate. It can even be caused by a digital rectal exam. For this reason, blood testing should always be done before and never after your exam.

Because false positive PSA results may lead to unnecessary testing (e.g., biopsies) and complications, there is controversy about whether the test should be used for routine screening. Some doctors prefer to monitor for increasing levels of PSA over time. Others will only order the study if there are symptoms present. Still others may choose not to order it at all. It is important that you have a discussion with your provider to discuss your options.

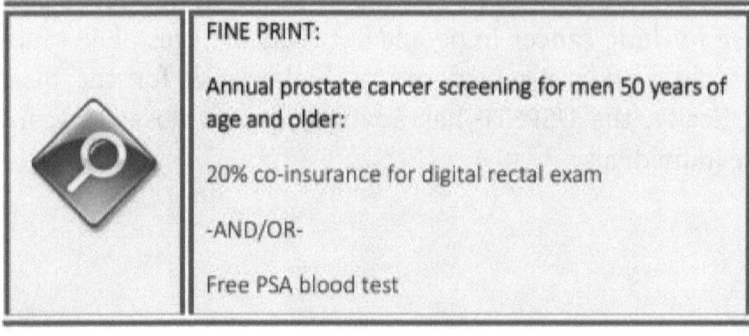

FINE PRINT:

Annual prostate cancer screening for men 50 years of age and older:

20% co-insurance for digital rectal exam

-AND/OR-

Free PSA blood test

Part B covers prostate cancer screening every 12 months. This may include a PSA screen covered free of charge or a digital rectal exam which requires a 20 percent co-insurance. The digital rectal exam allows your healthcare provider to actually feel the prostate to see if it is enlarged or has any suspicious masses on it suggestive for cancer.

Interestingly, the USPSTF does not make a formal statement regarding prostate cancer screening for men between the ages of 55 and 69 years of age. Instead, it is recommended that screening be pursued on an individual basis, based on a risk vs. benefit analysis between the patient and his doctor. The Task Force, however, outright advises against prostate cancer screening with a PSA test in men older than 70 years old. Medicare still covers testing for this age group.

Other Preventive Services

Lung cancer is the most common cancer affecting both men and women according to the CDC. In 2015, 218,527 people were diagnosed with lung cancer while nearly 153,718 died from the disease. It is the most common cause of cancer death for both men and women.

The USPSTF announced its recommendation in December 2013 to screen for lung cancer in people between the ages of 55- and 80-years old who are considered at higher risk for the disease. Specifically, the USPSTF has advised for low-dose CT scans in these individuals.

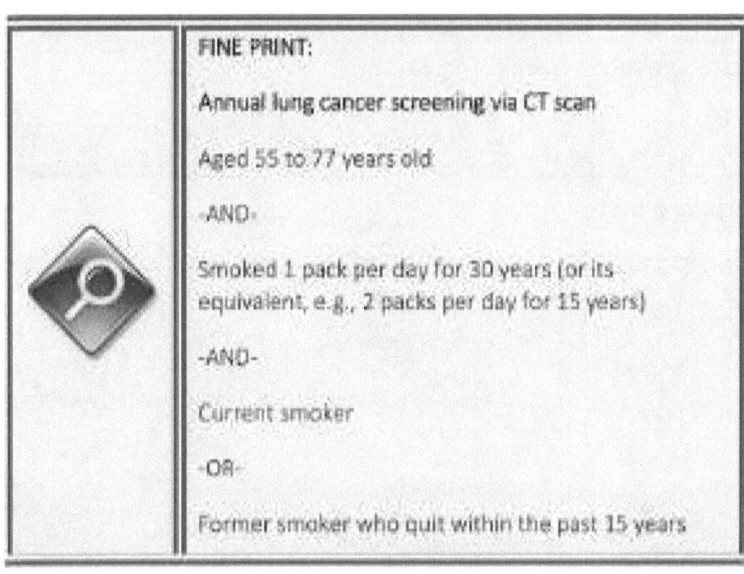

FINE PRINT:

Annual lung cancer screening via CT scan

Aged 55 to 77 years old

-AND-

Smoked 1 pack per day for 30 years (or its equivalent, e.g., 2 packs per day for 15 years)

-AND-

Current smoker

-OR-

Former smoker who quit within the past 15 years

In May 2014, Medicare declined to include these CT scans under its preventive care umbrella but later reversed its decision. As of February 2015, Medicare will now cover a low-dose CT scan once annually for current and past smokers if they quit within the past 15 years, if they are between the ages of 55 and 77 years old and if they smoked at least the equivalent of a pack of cigarettes a day for 30 years.

Concerns are being raised about the high rate of false-positive results. A 2017 study in JAMA Internal Medicine noted that nearly half of screening tests with low-dose CT scans in this population are positive but few are actually due to cancer. In fact, 97.5 percent of positive test results were confirmed to be false positives based on further and more invasive testing. Be sure to discuss the risk and benefits of screening with your doctor.

Osteoporosis is a disease that weakens bones and increases your risk for fracture and disability. According to the International Osteoporosis Foundation, 44 million Americans 50 and older have osteoporosis or low bone mass. Hip fractures hare associated with significant morbidity. As many as 20 to 24 percent of people will die in the first year after a hip fracture and their risk for death remains elevated over five years.

Part B covers screening of osteoporosis by way of bone density studies. These studies are covered every 24 months if certain risk criteria are met.

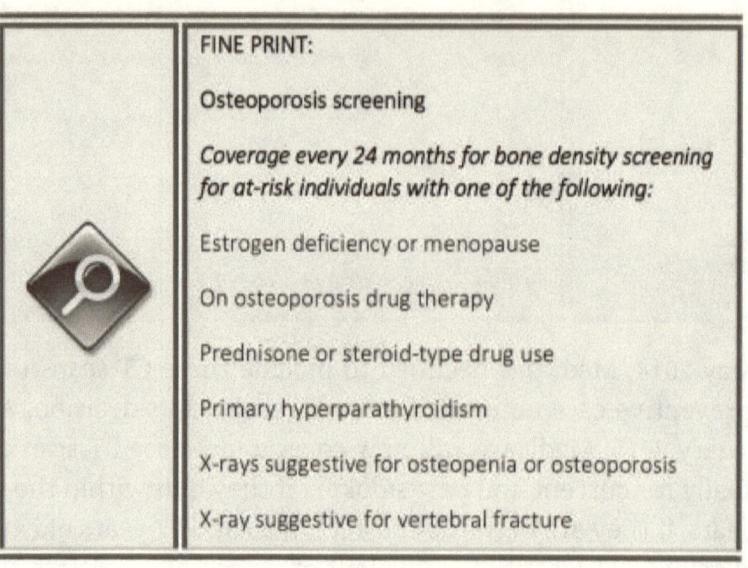

FINE PRINT:

Osteoporosis screening

Coverage every 24 months for bone density screening for at-risk individuals with one of the following:

Estrogen deficiency or menopause

On osteoporosis drug therapy

Prednisone or steroid-type drug use

Primary hyperparathyroidism

X-rays suggestive for osteopenia or osteoporosis

X-ray suggestive for vertebral fracture

For women, menopause is the most common cause. Estrogen generally protects the bones and when it decreases during menopause, the bones lose their strength. Other medical conditions that decrease estrogen will have a similar effect. Long-term use of steroid medications such as prednisone can also lead to thinning of the bones.

Hyperparathyroidism is a hormonal condition that may leech calcium out of bones, triggering osteoporosis. When x-rays suggest weakened bones or fractures of the vertebral spine, a bone density study may be indicated to confirm the diagnosis. Bone density studies may be required to monitor how well the bones are responding to treatments for osteoporosis.

Part B covers screening and counseling for other conditions as well. Tobacco use has serious health consequences ranging from heart disease to lung disease to cancer. The list goes on and on. Benefits of smoking cessation can be seen immediately as well as in the long-term.

Medicare recognizes the impact that smoking has on your health and offers coverage for eight one-on-one sessions of smoking cessation counseling over a 12-month period. These visits may review the consequences of smoking, an overview of behavioral interventions and considerations for medications to help you quit smoking, if appropriate. These visits come at a cost of a 20 percent co-insurance.

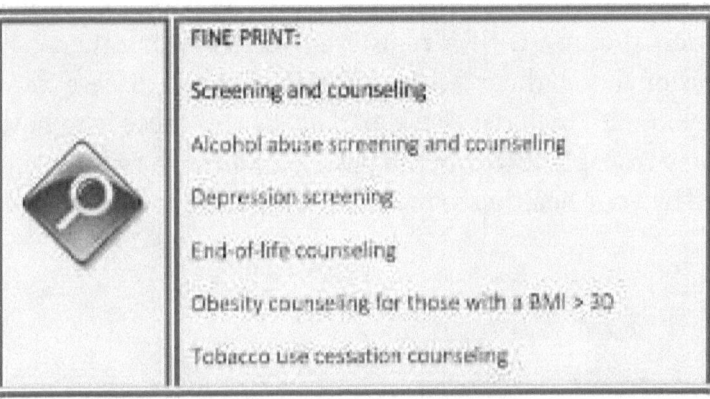

FINE PRINT:

Screening and counseling

Alcohol abuse screening and counseling

Depression screening

End-of-life counseling

Obesity counseling for those with a BMI > 30

Tobacco use cessation counseling

Alcohol overuse, similar to tobacco, can lead to an array of health complications, heart disease and liver disease to name a few. Steps taken to identify an abuse problem can help to mitigate these healthcare issues. Part B covers alcohol abuse counseling as a free preventive service annually.

Depression not only impairs quality of life but has been associated with heart disease. Part B covers annual depression screening free of charge once per year. In my opinion, healthcare providers should perform the screening as often as necessary without cost to the patient.

Obesity counseling is offered to those with a BMI greater than 30 without needing to pay. This may include discussions about diet, exercise and medical conditions that could be contributing to obesity. Behavioral modifications may be encouraged and the possibility of interventional medications reviewed.

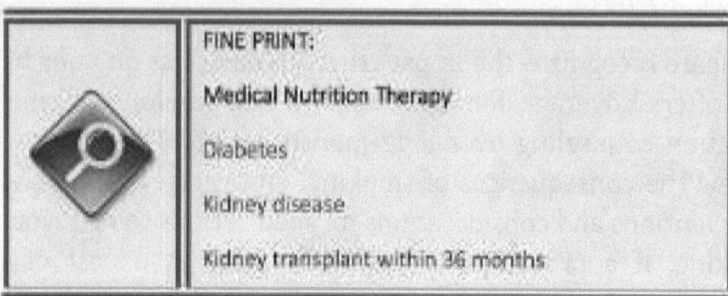

FINE PRINT:

Medical Nutrition Therapy

Diabetes

Kidney disease

Kidney transplant within 36 months

Medicare also covers one-on-one nutrition counseling or medical nutrition therapy with a registered dietician or other certified professional for those with diabetes, kidney disease or both. Kidney disease includes those on dialysis and those who have had a kidney transplant within the past 36 months. A referral must be placed by your healthcare provider for it to be covered.

What Your Provider Wishes Were Covered

I wish I could say that there were more preventive services offered through Medicare. The unfortunate truth is that the offerings, as good as they are, are limited. It may well be that your healthcare provider recommends additional tests and studies that Medicare may not cover based on your underlying conditions.

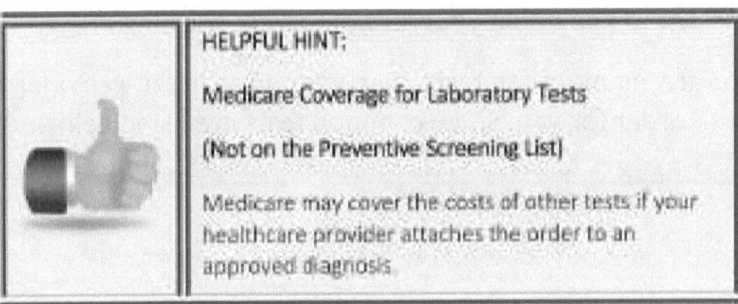

HELPFUL HINT:

Medicare Coverage for Laboratory Tests

(Not on the Preventive Screening List)

Medicare may cover the costs of other tests if your healthcare provider attaches the order to an approved diagnosis.

Throughout this book you have seen kidney disease mentioned time and again. Obviously, Medicare appreciates this to be a major health issue with serious consequences. The CDC estimates that 10 percent of Americans have some degree of chronic kidney disease and that risk for disease increases with age.

While certain factors may increase your risk for kidney disease, such as high blood pressure or diabetes, as much as 27 percent of kidney disease arises from other causes. Despite this fact, Medicare does not include blood tests to check your kidney function under its preventive services umbrella.

This does not mean that Medicare won't cover the tests at all. They may be covered if your healthcare provider attaches the order to a medical condition that you have. Some examples of approved diagnoses are diabetes and hypertension. As we have discussed in previous chapters, your healthcare provider must take care to select a Medicare-approved diagnosis code for that particular test or the costs will not be covered.

Kidney function is easily checked with simple and inexpensive blood tests. One of these is the serum creatinine test. According to the Healthcare Bluebook, the national average out-of-pocket cost for a serum creatinine test is $17. The test may be ordered on its own but is commonly included among a panel of tests, commonly referred to as chemistries or metabolic panels. Oddly enough, these panels are often less expensive than ordering the tests separately. If your healthcare provider does not offer one of these tests to you, I would encourage you to ask for it. It is very important to know that your kidneys are in working order.

There are many other tests that your healthcare provider may want to order for you. Some common tests are listed below.

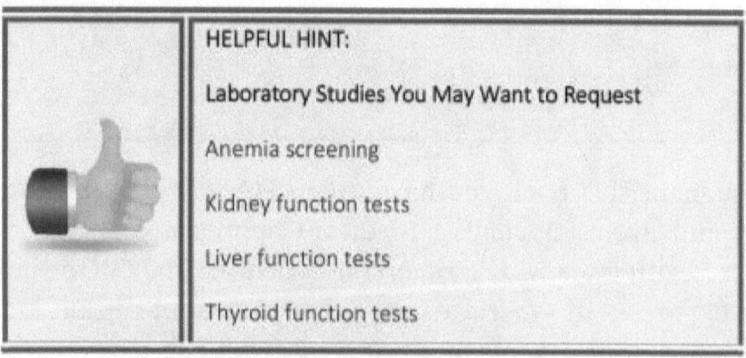

HELPFUL HINT:

Laboratory Studies You May Want to Request

Anemia screening

Kidney function tests

Liver function tests

Thyroid function tests

Anemia becomes all too common as we age for a variety of reasons, whether it be from malnutrition or a vitamin deficiency or even a warning sign that you are bleeding internally. Hemoglobin levels may be screened for directly with a $8 price tag or as part of a complete blood count for $21. Some offices even have a finger prick test that may cost you even less.

The liver is an essential organ that controls your metabolism. Knowing whether your liver is working appropriately is important, especially for those who take medications that must be processed by the liver. Liver function tests average $27 and a comprehensive metabolic panel, which includes liver function testing as well as kidney function, is $34.

A thyroid-stimulating hormone (TSH) test at $54 is used to screen for hypothyroidism, a condition that increases with age and that could result in abnormal heart rhythms, fatigue, and weight gain.

All of these costs are out-of-pocket expenses only if Medicare does not accept any of the cost responsibility. Again, if your provider attaches a diagnosis that Medicare approves for the test, you may have little or no cost.

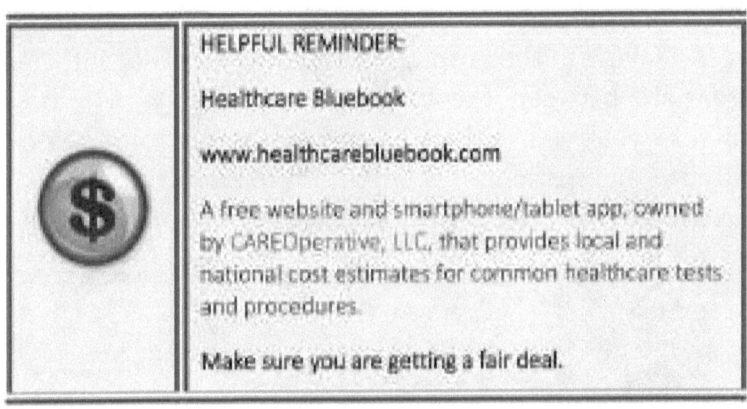

HELPFUL REMINDER:

Healthcare Bluebook

www.healthcarebluebook.com

A free website and smartphone/tablet app, owned by CAREOperative, LLC, that provides local and national cost estimates for common healthcare tests and procedures.

Make sure you are getting a fair deal.

What Defines an Inpatient?

What does it mean to be an inpatient? It may not be what you think. Even the dictionary does not know the full meaning of the word, at least not according to the Centers for Medicare and Medicaid Services (CMS).

There are two types of services you can be offered in the hospital. The first are outpatient services and the second are inpatient services. Staying in the hospital in and of itself is not sufficient to differentiate between the two. When you stay in a hospital overnight, you will either be placed under observation or admitted as an inpatient. It is important to know that observation services fall under the category of outpatient services.

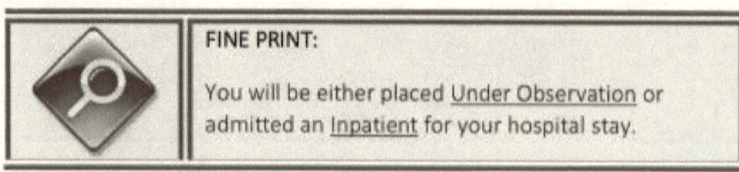

FINE PRINT:

You will be either placed Under Observation or admitted an Inpatient for your hospital stay.

How can you be under observation when you are actively being evaluated in the hospital? The doctor is already providing you care. CMS interprets this observation period as a time when a person can be monitored to see if they will require inpatient services. Inpatient care is ordered only when the medical concerns are considered urgent enough to require direct hospital care.

A simple way to look at the difference between the two services is to see that outpatient services can be performed at any time. Outpatient studies can be performed anywhere—in a doctor's office, a department in a hospital or any healthcare facility. These studies may provide important information but can be performed non-emergently.

Inpatient services require urgent evaluation for a condition that needs close supervision and monitoring. This may be a bit of an oversimplification but it relays the basic concept between outpatient and inpatient care.

Take the following example. A woman goes to see her doctor in the office about abdominal pain she had for several days. Her doctor suspects gallstones and orders an ultrasound. This is an outpatient study that can be performed in any Radiology department, whether that is in a hospital or not. He also orders some laboratory tests. She does not have to be admitted to the hospital to complete the evaluation. Her life is not at risk. If the doctor had concerns to this degree, he may have sent her to the hospital for a more urgent evaluation.

Another woman goes to the emergency room (ER) with the same symptoms. The ER doctor also suspects gallstones and orders laboratory studies and an ultrasound. If his concerns were for a severe or life-threatening condition, he may immediately admit her as an inpatient but often, until he has more information to guide his decision, he may place her under observation.

If the tests return negative, she may be sent home to follow-up with her doctor in an outpatient setting for further evaluation. If concerning findings are found, she may then be admitted as an inpatient for continued care. Again, this may be an oversimplification because in the brave new world of Medicare regulations, timing is everything.

The 2-Midnight Rule

On October 1, 2013, CMS implemented a change to Medicare that rocked hospital medicine to the core – the 2-Midnight Rule. The 2-Midnight Rule has drawn negative media coverage, vilifying doctors and hospitals to a fault. The fingers may be pointing in the wrong direction. Doctors and hospitals are equally unhappy about the change. The American Hospital Association has gone so far as to sue the federal government questioning the lawfulness of the act.

The 2-Midnight Rule can be summed up as follows: Medicare will not consider a patient's hospital stay appropriate for inpatient coverage unless it is expected to span two midnights. This requires one of two conditions:

The doctor documents and justifies that a hospital stay spanning two midnights is expected in the medical chart.

-OR-

The hospital stay actually crosses two midnights.

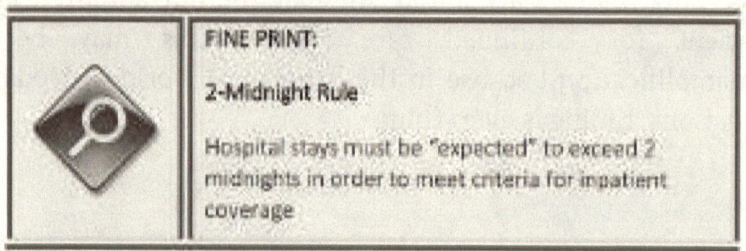

FINE PRINT:

2-Midnight Rule

Hospital stays must be "expected" to exceed 2 midnights in order to meet criteria for inpatient coverage

The two-midnight time stamp may seem arbitrary. By giving a formal definition, the government attempts to eliminate shades of grey about timing. Unfortunately, this definition has also added a degree of unfairness to hospital admissions. Someone admitted at 11:59am will cross two midnights almost 24 hours sooner than someone admitted two minutes later at 12:01am. With most hospitals entering orders electronically these days, there is no way to bypass that time stamp. That first patient, even if he requires the same exact care, may have a better opportunity to get inpatient coverage through Medicare.

Consider someone who has appendicitis. If a ruptured appendix is not removed, the patient could die. The medical services received in the hospital, appendectomy, are obviously medically necessary. Most people will go home the day after their appendix is removed. This patient would be deemed appropriate for observation services under the new ruling whereas they would have been considered inpatient-appropriate prior to the 2-Midnight Rule.

Other factors come into consideration when deciding how a patient should be admitted. A doctor needs to document his level of concern for the patient, which could potentially override the 2-Midnight Rule, though there is no guarantee that Medicare will accept the doctor's rationale for the admission.

The problem is that not all doctors document in the chart how long they expect a patient to stay in the hospital. Though they typically document a diagnosis and a care plan, doctors also need to write a statement that justifies why they think a patient is "expected" to stay more than two midnights. Without this documentation, the 2-Midnight Rule could remain unchallenged, with few exceptions.

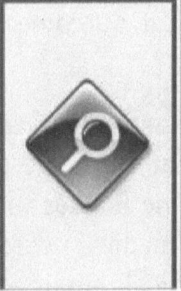

FINE PRINT:

Physician Documentation for Two Midnights

If a doctor documents a justifiable reason why a hospital stay is expected to exceed two midnights, he could potentially override the 2-Midnight Rule. There is no guarantee that Medicare will agree with the decision.

One would think that doctors could solve the two midnight conundrum by documenting a need for a two-midnight stay for all admissions. Even if the stay did not ultimately cross two midnights, Medicare may make an allowance based on the healthcare provider's documented concern.

Unfortunately, doing this across the board would constitute fraud. The consequences of a Medicare audit could destroy a healthcare provider's career and bankrupt hospitals. What the 2-Midnight Rule does is strip power from the healthcare provider. Their medical judgment is, to a certain extent, set aside in favor of an arbitrary timeline.

To be clear, the 2-Midnight Rule does NOT mean that if you stay in the hospital longer than 2 days you automatically become an inpatient. Medicare will only cover for inpatient services if they consider them medically necessary. Yes, there is another hoop to jump through.

Medical Necessity

Evidenced-based medicine is all the rage as well it should be. Evidence-based medicine favors using information from medical studies rather than long-held beliefs that may not have data to back them up. Evidence-based medicine aims to improve the quality of medical care and to improve clinical outcomes for patients.

Medicare's bent towards medical necessity is essentially a call to evidence-based medicine. The tricky part is that Medicare does not tell us exactly what evidence-based medicine it likes to use and does not spell out other rules that meet its medical necessity requirements. The reality is that every clinical situation is different and it can be difficult to decide whether or not a case meets Medicare inpatient criteria.

This is the reason why companies have developed strategies to help guide hospitals in their admissions processes. McKesson is a large corporation that has built a line of products known as InterQual®[4] to help medical providers and hospital systems make clinical decisions about patient cases. MCG Health provides a similar resource with their MCG™ Care Guidelines®[5]. InterQual and MCG Care Guidelines products are used by many managers and utilization reviewers across the country for use in their hospitals. You would be surprised by the subtle differences that can change a case from being appropriate for observation to being appropriate for inpatient status. Sometimes it is simply a matter of how fast IV fluid is being administered per hour.

Sometimes, however, even the most well-intentioned products will miss an inpatient case and call it appropriate for observation services. This is where a healthcare provider's medical judgment comes into play. Companies such as Executive Health Resources®[6] and R1 RCM®[7], formerly Accretive Health, offer case reviews by board-certified physicians across varied specialties. These physicians are trained in medical necessity compliance and assist hospitals in determining the appropriateness of inpatient admissions, according to available guidelines. Other companies may also provide similar services.

No method is perfect. Without full Medicare transparency on what they consider appropriate for inpatient criteria, even with InterQual or MCG Care Guidelines products and physician peer-to-peer reviews, there will always be a risk that Medicare will decline a claim. This can lead to appeals and months or years waiting for a judicial review.

Observation and Inpatient Costs

One has to ask whether it really makes a difference if you are under observation or admitted as an inpatient. Your wallet thinks so.

Someone admitted as an inpatient will have their hospital services covered by Medicare Part A. For every inpatient admission, there is a deductible of $1,340 that covers the first 60 days including hospital services, testing and medications. Medicare Part B services, however, will cover the physician fees. This requires the inpatient to pay a 20 percent co-insurance of the Medicare-approved cost for care provided by each medical provider.

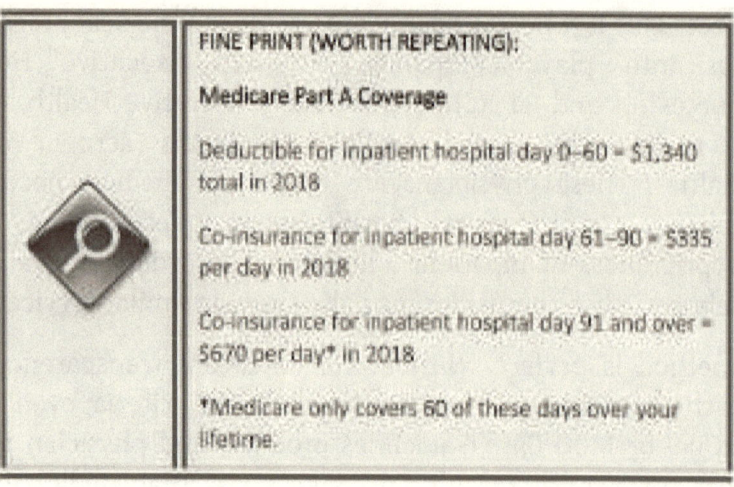

FINE PRINT (WORTH REPEATING):

Medicare Part A Coverage

Deductible for inpatient hospital day 0–60 = $1,340 total in 2018

Co-insurance for inpatient hospital day 61–90 = $335 per day in 2018

Co-insurance for inpatient hospital day 91 and over = $670 per day* in 2018

*Medicare only covers 60 of these days over your lifetime.

An individual placed under observation status will have his or her services covered by Medicare Part B, not Part A. Each service will be charged separately with a co-insurance or co-pay for each service. Physician services, as for inpatient status, will be billed at 20 percent of cost.

The good news is that a single co-pay cannot cost more than the $1,340 that your Medicare Part A deductible would have cost you. For example, if you undergo a specific procedure that costs $5,000, you will only be billed for $1,340.The bad news is that your services added up together can far exceed this amount.

FINE PRINT:

Medicare Part B Coverage

Whether you are placed under observation or are admitted as an inpatient, you will pay 20% of doctor fees.

Depending on your length of stay and the specific services provided, it may be far less expensive to be an inpatient. When you are under observation, Medicare saves money by shifting more of the costs to you. It does not mean that Medicare does not want you to be an inpatient. Medicare wants you to receive inpatient care when they deem it appropriate.

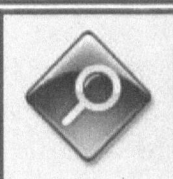

CONCEPT:

Hospitals tend to make less profit when you are placed under observation and would prefer you to be admitted as an inpatient.

To see how it plays out, let us use the example of appendicitis mentioned earlier in this chapter. According to Healthcare Bluebook, hospital services for a laparoscopic appendectomy average $9,000 to $10,000 nationwide over a two-day course. Additional days would be charged at $1,800 per day and shorter stays at a cost reduction of $1,800 per day.

Let's assume you have the surgery and stay in the hospital overnight for a two-day stay. If you are placed under observation, you would pay 20 percent of each service provided. That is 20 percent of the following (this list is not all-inclusive): anesthesia fees, imaging fees (e.g., CT scans), IV therapy, laboratory fees, medical/surgical supplies, operating room fees, pharmacy use, surgical fees, and room and board. Because Healthcare Bluebook does not break down the specifics of the hospital services, it is difficult to estimate how much you would really pay if you were under observation in this example. Regardless, when the costs are broken down, you will pay far more than the $1,340 you would have paid if you were admitted as an inpatient.

The sticker shock gets worse. These costs are only national estimates and Healthcare Bluebook warns that there can be as much as 400 percent variation depending on where the services are provided.

A hospital may even charge you differently based on whether you are under observation or admitted as an inpatient. To be honest, it is baffling that there would be any difference in cost for the same procedure.

A study published in the Archives of Internal Medicine in 2009 reviewed cost differences between 19,368 appendectomies in California. For individuals between the ages of 18- and 59-years old who stayed in the hospital less than 4 days, costs ranged from $1,500 to $180,000! The average cost was $33,000. The costs varied widely even within the same cities, despite no surgical complications in these cases.

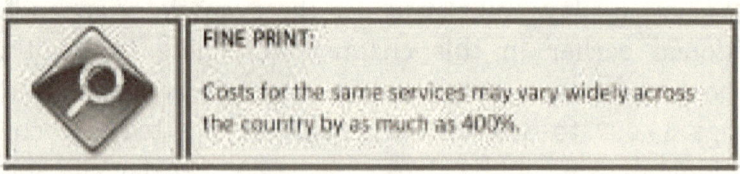

FINE PRINT:

Costs for the same services may vary widely across the country by as much as 400%.

California is not the only troublemaker state. A September 2013 report from the Obama administration found similar cost variation nationwide. The Centers for Medicare and Medicaid Services reviewed the costs of hospital stays across 3,000 healthcare facilities for the 100 most commonly billed diagnoses.

The differences were staggering. A joint replacement in Oklahoma cost $5,300 whereas one in Monterey, California cost $223,000. Admissions for congestive heart failure ranged from $21,000 to $46,000 in Denver, Colorado and between $9,000 to $51,000 in Jackson, Mississippi.

Of course, every patient situation is different but these cost differences are due to more than just particular health concerns. The system is rife with inequity.

Inpatient Only Surgeries

Even when you have surgery scheduled in advance, Medicare is not necessarily going to admit you as an inpatient. The Centers for Medicare and Medicaid Services has established a list of surgeries that will be covered by Medicare Part A while other surgeries, as long as there are no complications during the procedure, default to outpatient care under Medicare Part B coverage. The difference could cost you thousands of dollars.

Some surgeries that are not on the Inpatient Only List may be approved for inpatient care if the patient has significant risk factors that increase the likelihood for complications or that are expected to require a prolonged hospital stay for stabilization after surgery. These concerns must be documented in the medical chart by the surgeon who admits the patient. Otherwise, Medicare may not consider the surgery medically appropriate for an inpatient admission.

Every year CMS releases an updated version of the Inpatient Only List. The surgeries on this list are not arbitrarily selected. Due to the complexity of the procedure, the risk for complications, the need for post-operative monitoring, and an anticipated prolonged time for recovery, CMS understands that these surgeries require a high level of care. Examples of inpatient only surgeries include coronary artery bypass grafting, gastric bypass surgery, partial colectomy, and hip replacements.

In 2018, the controversial decision was made to take total knee arthroplasty, also known as a knee replacement, off the inpatient only list. According to CMS, 400,000 total knee and hip replacements were completed in 2014, costing Medicare $7 billion for hospitalizations relating to those procedures. This latest change to the Inpatient Only List is an obvious attempt to contain those costs. Unfortunately, by moving these surgeries from Part A to Part B, the cost is shifted to you, the patient.

FINE PRINT:

As of 2018, total knee replacements are no longer on the Inpatient Only List.

For the safety of Medicare beneficiaries, these surgeries must be performed in a hospital, not an ambulatory surgery center. Medicare Part A covers the majority of surgical costs with the $1,340 deductible.

Original Medicare and Medicare Advantage plans follow different rules. While Original Medicare follows the guidelines described above, Medicare Advantage plans do not have to. They can choose to pay for surgeries as inpatient or outpatient, i.e. pay more or less, regardless of their being on the Inpatient Only list. This could pose a financial hardship for you too.

Medications Received in the Hospital

Medications administered to an inpatient are covered under Part A. Medications given to someone under observation are a whole other story. These medications are considered to be "self-administered drugs". It is a bit of a misnomer as most of these medications will not be administered by the patient himself but by nursing staff.

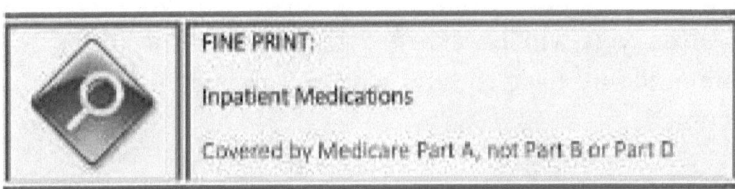

FINE PRINT:

Inpatient Medications

Covered by Medicare Part A, not Part B or Part D

In fact, for reasons of safety, the hospital rarely lets you bring in your own medications. The hospital cannot know with certainty that those medications are what you claim they are. It is not an issue of paranoia but one of liability. If something were to happen to you while taking one of these medications, the hospital could be at risk for not having provided you appropriate medication.

The hospital will usually provide you a medication in the same class if it does not have the specific one you take at home. If a medication does not have an alternative option available in the hospital pharmacy, the doctor may allow you to use your own medication if it is essential for your care. In order for someone to be able to use his own home medications, the provider must write specific orders on the chart allowing this to happen.

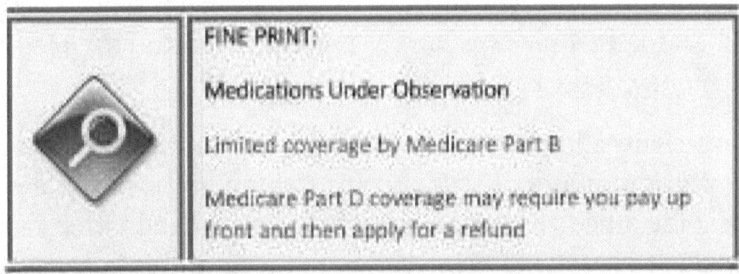

FINE PRINT:

Medications Under Observation

Limited coverage by Medicare Part B

Medicare Part D coverage may require you pay up front and then apply for a refund

The limited number of drugs that are covered under Medicare Part B will continue to be covered during an observation stay. You may remember that Part B pays toward certain IV medications administered by a licensed medical professional. For medications not covered under Part B, however, you will receive a bill for the full charges from the healthcare facility.

If you have Medicare Part D for prescription coverage, these drugs could potentially be covered. Hospital formularies are limited and may not match what is covered by your Part D plan. Most often you will be charged the cost of the drugs by the hospital and will have to send a claim to your Part D plan to get reimbursed.

MOON (Medicare Outpatient Observation Notice)

There is a lot of confusion about what the 2-Midnight Rule means. Some hospitals assume that after two midnights all cases are inpatient appropriate. Taken to an extreme, that assumption almost implies that hospitals should keep their patients in the hospital longer just so they can attain inpatient status.

There are so many things wrong with this. For one, this would add unnecessary days of care to a hospital stay and with that added costs. It makes healthcare less efficient and also decreases availability of resources to those who may need a hospital bed. The 2-Midnight Rule was surely not intended to cost Medicare more money in the end.

An inpatient admission is not based on time alone. Medical necessity comes into play. If you are staying in the hospital while waiting for a bed to become available in a rehabilitation facility or if you are receiving primarily nursing care, this is considered

112

custodial care. Medicare does not see custodial care as medically necessary. In their eyes, you could be receiving custodial care at another type of facility, whether it is a skilled nursing facility or in your own home. The intensity of care for these services is not high enough to meet criteria for an inpatient admission. Even if you are in the hospital for eight days, Medicare is not going to pay for an inpatient stay in this case.

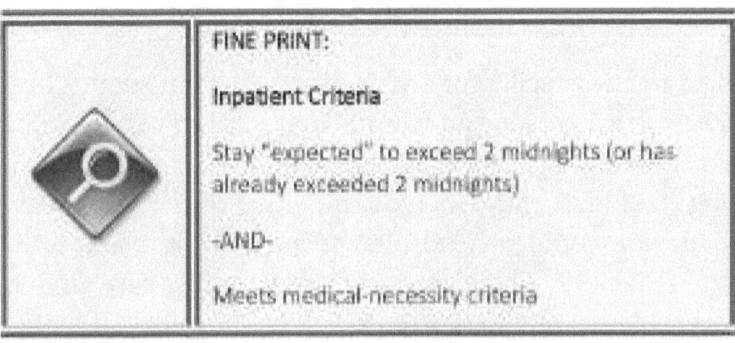

FINE PRINT:

Inpatient Criteria

Stay "expected" to exceed 2 midnights (or has already exceeded 2 midnights)

-AND-

Meets medical-necessity criteria

Ask your healthcare provider early on in the course of your hospital stay about your admission status. You may not be able to sway the doctor to admit you one way or the other. They have to do their job and base their orders on medical necessity. Healthcare providers risk being audited by Medicare otherwise and those audits could have consequences on their career.

You have a right to know whether you are being admitted as an inpatient or placed under observation. In fact, the hospital must provide you with a Medicare Outpatient Observation Notice (MOON) if you have received 24 or more hours of observation care and they must do so within 36 hours of a healthcare provider writing an observation order. Specifically, the MOON will notify you that you are not an inpatient and will list the reasons why.

Your being aware of your inpatient vs. observation status is important as you should be involved in decisions on how much testing should be allowed under the circumstances. Costs may be a big factor for you to consider.

Skilled Nursing, Hospice &

Medicare

Skilled Nursing Facilities (SNF)

A skilled nursing facility or SNF is exactly what it sounds like. It is a place where a person can be provided nursing care from people with qualified skills and medical expertise. Examples of skilled nursing facilities may include qualified nursing homes and rehabilitation centers. A hospital technically is also a SNF. You stay in a facility where you receive nursing care and more. However, Medicare chooses to categorize hospitals in a different way. Hospitals are acute care facilities and are considered a higher level of care than a SNF.

Despite the distinction between a hospital and a SNF, Medicare Part A is the part of Medicare that provides coverage for both. We discussed the terms for hospital inpatient coverage in Chapter 7 but a whole new set of rules are put in place for care beyond those hospital walls.

What Counts as Skilled Care?

For Medicare to cover a SNF admission, it must see that skilled care is required on a daily basis. That care must be ordered by a healthcare provider. For the purposes of Medicare, your care is considered daily even if the therapy services are offered only 5 or 6 days a week.

To be considered skilled care, the services must be performed or supervised by trained professionals. In addition to physicians, physician assistants and advanced practice nurse practitioners, other qualifying professionals include audiologists, occupational therapists, speech-language pathologists, physical therapists and registered nurses.

FINE PRINT:

Skilled services must be offered at least 5 days per week to meet criteria for a Medicare approved SNF stay.

The skilled services covered by Medicare include the following:

- Occupational Therapy services
- Physical Therapy services
- Skilled nursing care
- Speech-Language Pathology services

Custodial care alone is not considered sufficient for Medicare coverage. For example, some patients may need assistance in bathing, dressing, toileting and managing colostomy bags or urinary catheters. Some may need help getting in and out of bed while others may need help in feeding and taking their medications or supplying their oxygen. All of these activities are important to the care of the patient but fall under custodial care.

These services are offered in nursing homes but alone do not meet the level of acuity required for Medicare Part A coverage.

Other items covered by Medicare for people who are admitted to a SNF would include:

- Ambulance transportation to other healthcare facilities as medically necessary

- Dietary counseling

- Meals

- Medical supplies and equipment

- Medications

- Meals

- Semi-private room (you may have to share a room)

- Social service

Skilled Nursing facility Timelines

Keeping all the different Medicare timelines straight can be quite a chore. There are timelines needed to qualify for SNF coverage. Medicare will not cover a stay in a SNF unless you are first admitted to a hospital as an inpatient. Chapter 7 showed us the complexities of the inpatient admission process. Transferring to a SNF after that hospital stay is even more complicated.

Not only must you be admitted as an inpatient but you must be admitted as an inpatient for three consecutive days in order to qualify for coverage. To complicate things, the day you are discharged from the hospital does not count as one of the required three inpatient days. This means you must have been in the hospital for four days. Any days that you were placed under observation status do not count towards the requirement.

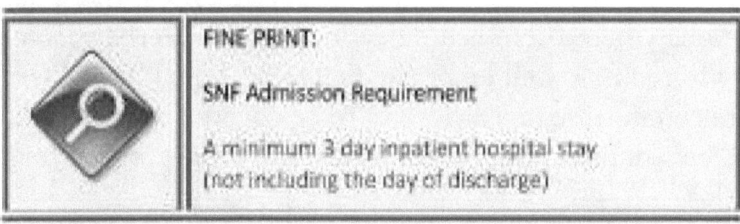

FINE PRINT:

SNF Admission Requirement

A minimum 3 day inpatient hospital stay (not including the day of discharge)

The three-day inpatient hospital requirement for skilled nursing facility care may not necessarily apply if you are on a Medicare Advantage plan. These plans, run by private insurance companies, have the option not to participate in this particular rule.

From a business point of view, Original Medicare uses the rule to make sure it only pays for skilled nursing facility care for those people who have demonstrated the most serious illness. The rulings also aims to decrease the odds that a patient would be discharged from the hospital prematurely. By assuring that patients receive proper services before they are transferred to a SNF, the risk for a subsequent inpatient hospitalization, referred to as a readmission, is reduced.

Medicare Advantage plans have a different approach. If a patient is likely to be transferred to a skilled nursing facility in any case, it is in the insurance company's best interest financially to transfer the patient from the more expensive hospital to the less expensive skilled nursing facility as soon as possible. A 2015 study in Health Affairs found that waiving the three-day requirement was medically safe. Not only were people no less likely to be readmitted to the hospital when the rule was waived but their stays in the skilled nursing facility were of a similar duration as people who were subjected to the three-day requirement. Simply put, leaving the hospital earlier did not cause patients to stay longer in a skilled nursing facility.

Once the three-day criteria is met, there is a limited window on which you can be admitted into the SNF. Most people will be directly admitted to the SNF from the hospital but there may be situations where there is a delay in SNF care. Perhaps someone wants to see how well he or she does with home health services before committing to a SNF stay. To be covered by Medicare, you must be admitted to the SNF within 30 days of leaving the hospital.

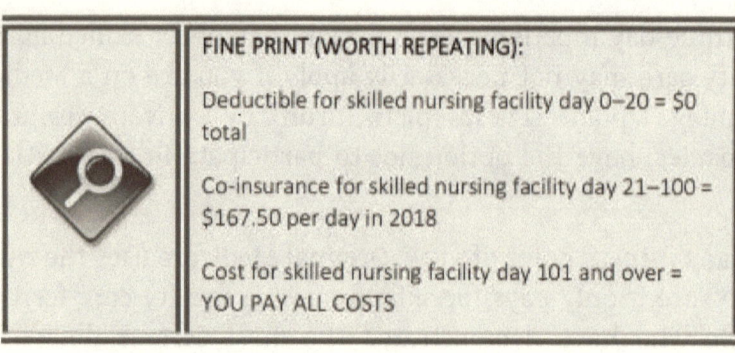

FINE PRINT (WORTH REPEATING):

Deductible for skilled nursing facility day 0–20 = $0 total

Co-insurance for skilled nursing facility day 21–100 = $167.50 per day in 2018

Cost for skilled nursing facility day 101 and over = YOU PAY ALL COSTS

Medicare will cover the first 20 days of your SNF stay at no charge and the next 80 days at $167.50 per day. After that you are on your own. Medicare may cover costs for up to 100 days but your benefit window is only 60 days. This is where things get confusing.

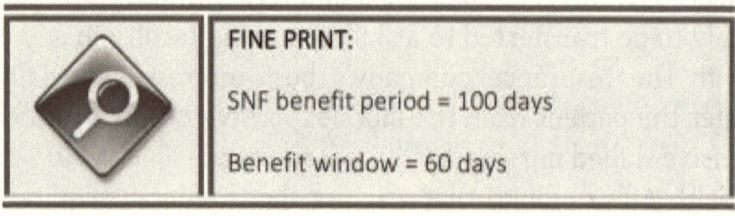

FINE PRINT:

SNF benefit period = 100 days

Benefit window = 60 days

Medicare may stop paying for SNF care for a number of reasons. You may leave a SNF because your condition is fully resolved. Once you are stable, you may choose to leave a SNF and pursue home health services instead. It could also be that while you are at a nursing home, skilled nursing care is stopped. That level of care may no longer be needed but custodial care may continue for your basic day-to-day living.

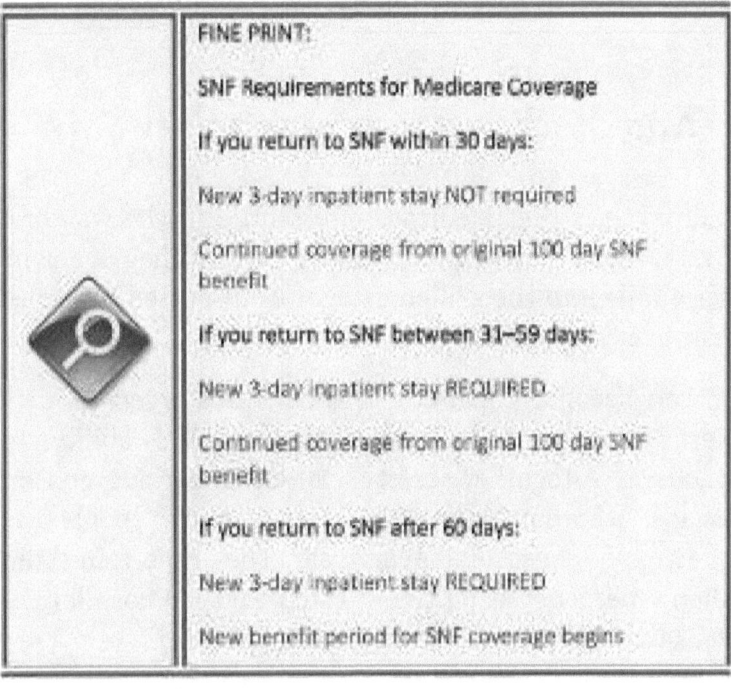

FINE PRINT:

SNF Requirements for Medicare Coverage

If you return to SNF within 30 days:

New 3-day inpatient stay NOT required

Continued coverage from original 100 day SNF benefit

If you return to SNF between 31–59 days:

New 3-day inpatient stay REQUIRED

Continued coverage from original 100 day SNF benefit

If you return to SNF after 60 days:

New 3-day inpatient stay REQUIRED

New benefit period for SNF coverage begins

Life is never predictable. Your medical condition may deteriorate and you may again need skilled nursing care. This is when your benefit window comes into play. If you return to a SNF (any SNF, not necessarily the one where you originally stayed) within 30 days, Medicare will continue its coverage as if you never left the facility. Any remaining days from the original SNF 100-day coverage period will then be used.

If you return to the SNF between 31 and 59 days from your SNF stay, Medicare will require that you have a new three-day inpatient hospital admission. Your current coverage window would continue. Any days already used would count toward the 100 days of coverage.

If you return to the SNF 60 days or later, again you will require a new three-day inpatient hospital admission but you will start a new benefit and coverage period, starting with SNF day #0.

Non-Medicare Nursing Facility Stays

The sad truth is that Medicare offers little in the way of long-term care. Many people need nursing care as they age, whether that care falls into the skilled categories discussed previously or for basic everyday needs.

Vision can become impaired. Balance issues creep in for some people. Cognitive decline can impact one's ability to be independent. Altogether, safety can be a serious concern as people age. According to the CDC, one out of four people over the age of 65 experiences a fall every year. They report an estimated 3 million emergency department visits, 800,000 hospitalizations, and 28,000 deaths from falls each year.

FACT CHECK:

1 in 4 people over the age of 65 experiences a fall every year

With many people likely to need help with the activities of daily living as they get older, many may have to turn to nursing homes for care. Unfortunately, long-term stays in a nursing home are not covered by Medicare.

The costs of nursing home care can be staggering. In 2017, the average cost for a semi-private or shared room was $7,148 per month. That's $85,766 per year A private room cost more at $8,121 per month, or $97,452 per year!

Some private insurance plans may offer coverage for nursing home stays through a managed care plan or long-term care insurance. For these private plans, a contract agreement between the insurance company and the specific nursing home is needed for you to be provided coverage.

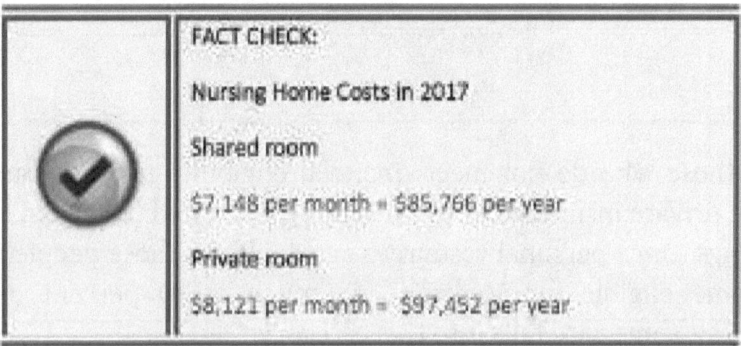

FACT CHECK:

Nursing Home Costs in 2017

Shared room

$7,148 per month = $85,766 per year

Private room

$8,121 per month = $97,452 per year

From my experience, you may be hard-pressed to find an insurance plan that covers enough of the needed services without being subject to an exorbitant monthly premium. Also, these plans are unlikely to cover the entire cost of the nursing home stay, which adds more monthly fees for you to pay.

A more common option for many people is to default to Medicaid. Medicaid offers healthcare services to Americans with low incomes. It is funded on federal and state levels but run by state governments. For this reason, eligibility for Medicaid will vary state by state. With resistance from certain states to implement certain provisions of the Affordable Care Act, Medicaid coverage remains a bit unpredictable at this time. Medicaid may allow for nursing home coverage at certified, government-approved, nursing homes.

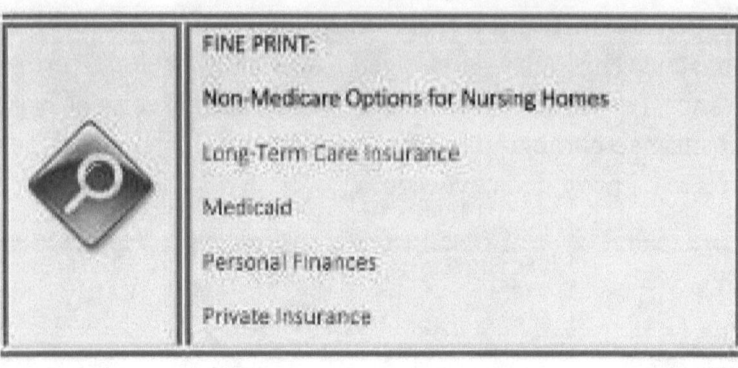

For those who do not meet financial eligibility for Medicaid or have private insurance, they most likely will need to rely on their savings. Once personal resources are depleted, those people may become eligible for Medicaid. As much as 60 percent of all nursing home care falls into this category.

It is in your best interest to reach out to an elder law attorney if you have concerns about Medicaid. For obvious reasons, many people hope to preserve their assets for their spouse, children, and future generations. An attorney may be able to address different options from estate planning to "Medicaid trusts" that can help address your financial situation.

End-of-Life Counseling

End-of-life counseling is a new benefit offered to beneficiaries as of 2016. These counseling sessions are free of charge and allow time for people to discuss their medical options and long-term wishes with their healthcare providers.

End-of-life counseling may be helpful for beneficiaries dealing with serious chronic medical conditions and worse, terminal conditions. These are not "death panels" and they are not mandatory. Anyone can change their minds about their care plans at any time. The intent is to allow adequate time to address and educate around this important issue.

Hospice Care

Long-term care at a nursing home is one thing but end-of-life care is another. Hospice is end-of-life care provided by qualified professionals to assist you and your family through a terminal illness.

These can be challenging times, both emotionally and physically, and a team of hospice-trained individuals will be available to ease your transition. This team may include physicians, nurse practitioners, nurses, counsellors, occupational therapists, physical therapists, speech-language pathologists, social workers, hospice aides and volunteers. A doctor who specializes in hospice care will be assigned to you but you may also receive care from your regular primary care provider. A hospice nurse and physician will be on-call for you 24 hours a day 7 days a week.

Once a physician certifies that an individual is terminally ill and expected to live less than 6 months, that individual becomes eligible for Hospice care. This is very important. Medicare requires that a physician make this certification, not any other type of licensed provider. After the initial certification is made, another healthcare provider, i.e., an advanced practice nurse practitioner or a physician assistant, may step in as the primary caregiver if preferred by the patient.

As we all know, doctors are not God. At best, the doctor can only use statistical estimates as a point of reference. We are all unique. These estimates may be too short or too long. What these life expectancies allow is for people to make their end-of-life plans if they so choose.

Some people become angry when a doctor tells them how much longer they may have to live. I can assure you no doctor likes to do it. It is an uncomfortable and often dreary discussion. The doctor is only trying to provide you information about the limited options to treat your condition. You, not the doctor, are the one who decides how to use that information.

Many people hope to prove the doctor wrong by living long past the deadline. Good for them! For the purposes of Hospice care, 6 months or less is the amount of time you are expected to live before Medicare will pay for services.

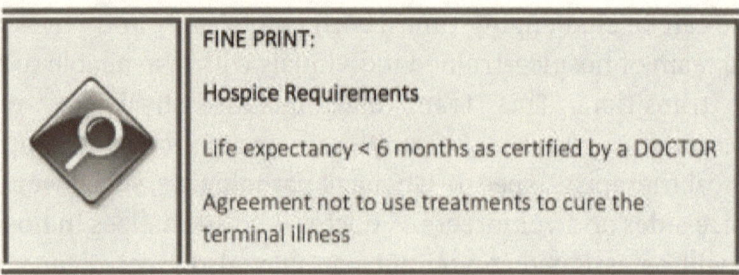

FINE PRINT:

Hospice Requirements

Life expectancy < 6 months as certified by a DOCTOR

Agreement not to use treatments to cure the terminal illness

Once a terminal diagnosis is made, Hospice care may be pursued if a decision is made to forego treatments that would attempt to cure the condition. For example, someone on Hospice would not be allowed to have chemotherapy to treat cancer if that cancer was the diagnosis that put him in Hospice in the first place. Chemotherapy would be an attempted treatment to cure the condition.

Your healthcare provider may have tried treatments that did not work or may find that the harms and side effects of other treatments may outweigh the benefits. Whatever the case may be, choosing Hospice care is a thoughtful decision to be made between the healthcare provider and his patient. Families are often involved in these complex decisions. I encourage family meetings with the provider to discuss the issues involved in making an informed choice.

Hospice care may be provided in your home or a Medicare-approved hospice facility, hospital hospice unit, or nursing home.

What Hospice Does (Not) Cover

Becoming a Hospice patient does not mean that all care is cut off. Palliative care, or comfort care, will allow symptom relief to ease any pain or suffering. Hospice provides an array of services to the patient including doctor services, dietary counselling, grief counselling, homemaker services, medical supplies and equipment, medications for comfort care, nursing care, Occupational Therapy, Physical Therapy, Social Work services and Speech-Language Pathology services.

Hospice may also allow for inpatient stays if needed for comfort care, i.e., pain and symptom control for the terminal condition. Respite care is a placement option that may offer relief for those caring for the patient in the home. Both of these are provided as short-term options only and must be approved and arranged by the Hospice team for Medicare to pay. Medicare covers respite services but requires a 5 percent co-insurance.

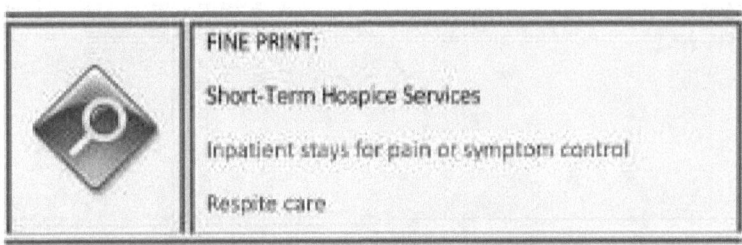

FINE PRINT:

Short-Term Hospice Services

Inpatient stays for pain or symptom control

Respite care

There may be times when a condition other than the terminal illness requires medical attention. For example, a urinary tract infection could cause unnecessary discomfort or even lead to complications with bacteria getting into the blood stream. Emergency room and even hospital care may be needed to treat and cure the condition. In this case, antibiotics would definitively treat the infection.

Original Medicare (Part A and Part B) may cover these services but it is best that you contact your hospice team before pursing treatment. The team will determine officially whether the condition is related to your terminal illness. You do not want to lose your Hospice benefits if you receive treatments that do not meet criteria.

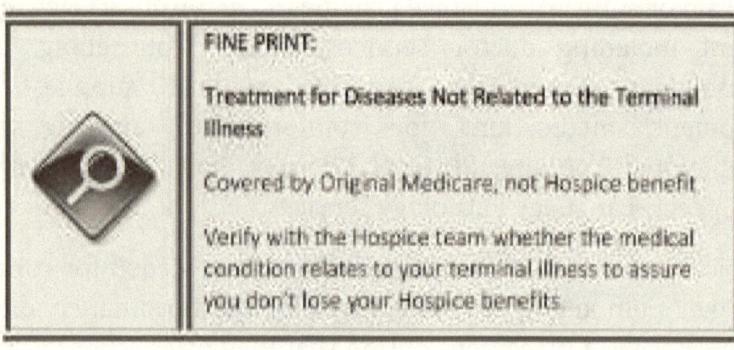

FINE PRINT:

Treatment for Diseases Not Related to the Terminal Illness

Covered by Original Medicare, not Hospice benefit

Verify with the Hospice team whether the medical condition relates to your terminal illness to assure you don't lose your Hospice benefits

Medicare, however, will not cover medications or treatments intended to cure your terminal condition. If new treatments become available or your condition changes, you may consider stopping Hospice care to pursue these options. Care from a provider not on or approved by your Hospice team will also not be covered.

Logistics of Hospice

To be enrolled in Hospice, you must have both Medicare Part A and Part B benefits. The monthly premiums, deductibles, co-pays and co-insurance apply as for all other Medicare-covered services as discussed in Chapter 3.

Hospice services are covered by Medicare Part A. The majority of Hospice services are covered with the following exceptions:

- Room and board is not covered whether you are at home or in a Medicare-approved Hospice facility. This does not include inpatient hospital stays approved by the Hospice team.

- Medications for pain and symptom control may require a co-pay up to $5 when you are at home. Medicare covers inpatient medications.

- Respite care requires a 5 percent co-insurance of the Medicare-approved amount.

Hospice is broken down into a series of benefit periods. The first two periods are at 90 day intervals. Subsequent benefit periods start every 60 days. A doctor must certify that you have a terminal illness at the start of each benefit period. As you can see, Hospice care can extend long after the initial expected 6-month interval.

Doctors can't see into the future. They can only use statistics to give an estimate about someone's life expectancy. The 6-month life expectancy is what makes you initially eligible for Hospice care in the first place.

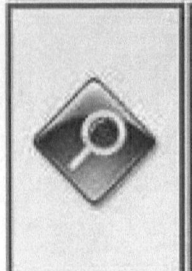

FINE PRINT:

Hospice Benefit Periods

Two 90-day benefit periods

Then 60-day benefit periods until Hospice care ends

Option to change providers once per benefit period

The benefit periods allow Medicare to confirm that you have a terminal illness and that coverage should continue. They also allow you an opportunity to change your healthcare providers if you want. You can only do this once during each benefit period.

CHOOSING THE RIGHT MEDICARE

PLAN

When Should You Decline Medicare

If you don't need Medicare, you can always decline it, right? Be careful before you make that decision. There could be serious consequences.

Part A is funded by the Medicare Trust Fund. You paid payroll taxes to earn that benefit, just like you paid taxes toward Social Security. If you paid at least 40 quarters of Medicare taxes, your Part A premiums are offered to you at no cost.

Declining Part A when you are receiving Social Security benefits of any kind is problematic. Why? Because not only will you lose access to Part A, but your Social Security benefits will come to a screeching halt too. This is especially important to note if you are receiving retirement benefits or are on Social Security Disability Insurance (SSDI).

After someone has been on SSDI for 24 months, they become eligible for Medicare. Declining Part A, a tax-earned benefit, will also end their disability benefits, also a taxed-earned benefit. Ultimately, they end up without income or health coverage!

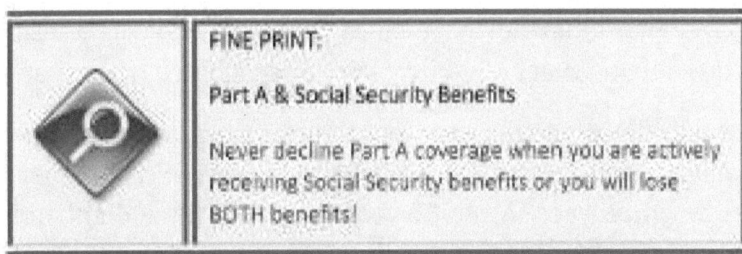

FINE PRINT:

Part A & Social Security Benefits

Never decline Part A coverage when you are actively receiving Social Security benefits or you will lose BOTH benefits!

Why would you want to decline Medicare in the first place?

- You already have employer-sponsored coverage and do not want to pay for two premiums.

- You could get cheaper health care from the Health Insurance Marketplace or elsewhere.

- You want to take advantage of a health savings account (HSA).

Employer-sponsored health plans do not all work the same way. Some of them will require that you sign up for Medicare when you become eligible. If you don't, they could refuse coverage. This is because they want Medicare to pay first and they intend to pay whatever is left over. Other employers may end your healthcare benefits if you sign up for Medicare!

Please reach out to your employer to find out how their health plan works with Medicare.

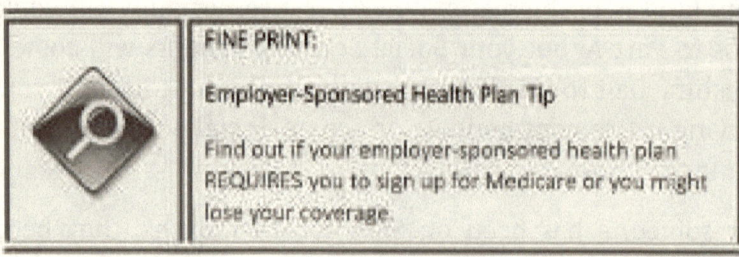

FINE PRINT:

Employer-Sponsored Health Plan Tip

Find out if your employer-sponsored health plan REQUIRES you to sign up for Medicare or you might lose your coverage.

Of course, no one wants to pay more than they have to. Paying premiums for both an employer-sponsored plan and Medicare can cost a bundle. It is reasonable to defer Medicare if your employer plan does not have rules that require it otherwise but only do so if you meet eligibility for a Special Enrollment Period.

As a reminder, Special Enrollment Periods are offered to people who have health coverage from an employer that hires at least 20 full-time employees. After 65 years old, you have eight months from the time you lose that health coverage or you leave that job, whichever comes first, to sign up for Medicare. Without this Special Enrollment Period, you could face late penalties that could last as long as you have Medicare. In the end, you could pay more overall than if you paid the premiums for both the employer-sponsored health plan and Medicare in the first place.

Another penalty of declining Medicare relates more to timing than money. If you miss your Initial Enrollment Period or Special Enrollment Period, or if you decline Medicare but later decide you want to enroll, when can you sign up? There is a General Enrollment Period that occurs every year from January 1 to March 31. You apply during this time but your Medicare benefits will not begin until July 1. That is a long time to be without health insurance! In fact, if you lose access to your other health plan while waiting for Medicare benefits, you could be left without coverage anywhere from 3 to 14 months.

Medicare may not always be your cheapest option but it is usually your best bet. You may find that a Health Insurance Marketplace Plan or another plan has a lower premium or deductible compared to Medicare. However, if you are on Medicare, you are not eligible for these plans. It is actually against the law for an insurer to offer you one. If you decline Medicare in favor of one of these other plans, you will face late penalties when you sign up for Medicare later. This will likely cost you more in the long run.

Some people benefit from health savings accounts (HSA) but at the time of this publication that benefit stops once you accept Medicare. An HSA is a tax-sheltered medical savings account used to pay for healthcare expenses for people who have high-deductible insurance plans. You can no longer add money to your HSA once you are on Medicare, though you can continue to use what already funds are in the account towards qualifying medical expenses. That being the case, once the money dries up, so does your access to an HSA.

The GOP 2019 Fiscal Year Budget proposed that Medicare beneficiaries be allowed to set aside money tax-free for the purposes of paying for healthcare expenses. It would also make the cost of premiums tax deductible (an amount ranging from $1,791 to $5,326 for Medicare Part B in 2018). How wonderful it would be if seniors could save more of their retirement earnings! Although the budget did not pass, it is a hopeful sign of Medicare changes to come.

Where Does Medigap Fit In?

Before you decide whether or not you want to go with Original Medicare or a Medicare Advantage plan, you need to understand what options are available to supplement your coverage.

Medigap plans, as discussed in Chapter 2, are Medicare Supplement Insurance plans offered by private insurance companies that can help you to pay for deductibles, co-insurance, and other fees left uncovered by Original Medicare.

Medigap plans are lettered alphabetically from A to N but do not confuse them with the "parts" of Medicare, i.e., A, B, C and D. Medigap plans are NOT officially a part of the Medicare program.

These lettered plans are standardized by the federal government and are the same across all states with the exceptions of Massachusetts, Minnesota, and Wisconsin which offer their own variations. Minnesota, while offering its own state plan, does also offer the F (high-deductible version), K, L, M, and N plans.

All insurance companies must offer at least Plan A and either Plan C or F. Take note that Plans E, H, I, and J are no longer available. Some plans have high deductibles to pay before benefits kick in. These include plan K with a $5,240 deductible and plan L with a $2,620 deductible in 2018. Plan F has an original version and also a high-deductible version which requires you to pay $2,240 out of pocket for coverage with the exception of foreign travel which requires an additional $250 deductible.

Medicare SELECT plans are an alternative to Medigap plans in certain states. These plans are generally less expensive than Medigap plans but for good reason. Medicare SELECT plans are limited to a network of providers and will not pay toward any services provided out of that network.

Signing up for Medigap is the tricky part. You have a 6-month Open Enrollment Period (which really ought to be called an Initial Enrollment Period) that begins the day you enroll in Medicare Part B. Your Medigap coverage begins on the first day of the month after you apply.

If you apply late for Medigap, the private insurance company can refuse or deny coverage to you based on medical conditions you have at the time of your application. These are referred to as pre-existing conditions. You may even have to wait six months before Medigap benefits begin if you have certain medical conditions.

Summary of Medigap Plan Benefits in 2018

	A	B	C	D	F	G	K	L	M	N
Part A Deductible		•	•	•	•	•	50%	75%	50%	•
Part A Hospice Co-insurance	•	•		•	•	•	50%	75%	•	•
Part A Hospital Co-insurance up to 365 Days after Medicare Benefits Are Used Up	•	•	•	•	•	•	•	•	•	•
Part A SNF Co-insurance			•	•	•	•	50%	75%	•	•
Part B Deductible			•		•					
Part B Co-insurance	•	•	•	•	•	•	50%	75%	•	•
Part B Excess Charges					•	•				
First 3 Pints of Blood	•	•	•	•	•	•	50%	75%	•	•
Foreign Travel			80%	80%	80%	80%			80%	80%

State Specific Medigap Plan Benefits in 2018

	Massachusetts	Minnesota	Wisconsin
Part A Deductible	Supplemental Plan only	Extended Basic Plan only	Available in certain plans
Part A Hospital Co-insurance	•	•	•
Part A Hospice	•	•	•
Part A Inpatient Mental Health Stays	60 days (120 days for Supplemental Plan)		175 days after Medicare exhausted
Part A SNF Co-insurance	Supplemental Plan only	100 days (120 days for Extended Basic Plan)	•
Part B Deductible	Supplemental Plan only	Extended Basic Plan only	Available in certain plans
Part B Co-insurance	•	•	Available in certain plans
First 3 Pints of Blood	•	•	•
Foreign Travel Emergency	Supplemental Plan only	80%	Available in certain plans
Home Health Services			40 visits (may increase up to 365 visits with certain plans)

If you apply for a Medigap plan outside of the Open Enrollment Period, you may still be offered some protection against medical underwriting for pre-existing conditions but only if you meet one of the following criteria:

- Your Medicare Advantage plan is no longer available to you and you want to change to Original Medicare.

- You want to switch from a Medicare Advantage plan to Original Medicare within the first 12 months of your initial eligibility.

- You lose access to a non-Medicare supplemental policy, e.g., an employer-sponsored health plan or COBRA coverage.

- You lose access to your Medicare SELECT plan due to relocation.

- You want to switch back to a Medigap plan after switching from a Medigap plan to a Medicare Advantage Plan.

- Your Medigap plan ends through no fault of your own.

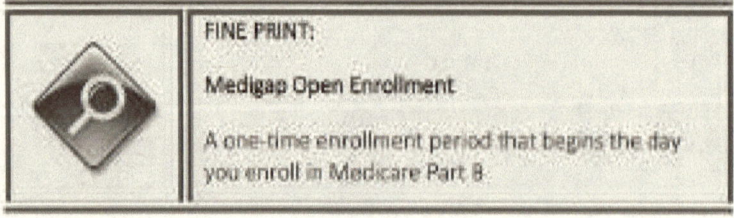

FINE PRINT:

Medigap Open Enrollment

A one-time enrollment period that begins the day you enroll in Medicare Part B

Take note that not all states offer Medigap plans to Medicare beneficiaries who are younger than 65 years old.

Travel with Medicare, Medicare Advantage

and Medigap

One of the biggest fees often left uncovered by Medicare is health care when you travel out of the country. That may be an issue if you are someone who hopes to travel the world when you retire.

Original Medicare will only pay for emergency health care in a foreign country when:

- You receive care in a foreign hospital because it is closer than an American one, even if you are in the United States when the medical emergency occurs.

- You receive care in a foreign hospital that is closer to your home than an American hospital.

- You receive care in a Canadian hospital when traveling directly between Alaska and the contiguous United States.

- You are on a cruise ship within six hours of a U.S. port or U.S. territory waters.

If you travel a lot, a Medigap plan may be something to consider. The plans that offer travel coverage (plans C, D, F, G, and N) will pay up to 80 percent of any emergency care you receive. However, they will only do so for the first 60 days you are out of the country. The clock resets after you return to the United States.

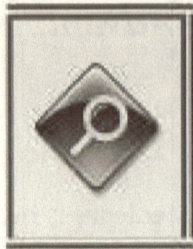

FINE PRINT:

Foreign Travel

Original Medicare does not usually cover health care received in foreign countries but some Medigap plans do.

Another alternative is to find a Medicare Advantage plan that also offers coverage options for foreign travel.

Choosing Between Medigap and Medicare

Advantage

Medigap plans are not part of Original Medicare though they can be used together with Original Medicare to, hopefully, save you money. What you cannot do is supplement a Medicare Advantage plan with a Medigap plan.

Knowing whether or not you will save more or get better care using a Medigap plan or a Medicare Advantage plan is not always easy. Everyone has different budgets and healthcare needs.

For some people the choice between Medigap and Medicare Advantage is easy, and in some cases, the decision is already made for you. Some states do not offer Medigap policies to people younger than 65 years old. You also cannot be on a Medigap plan if you are also on Medicaid.

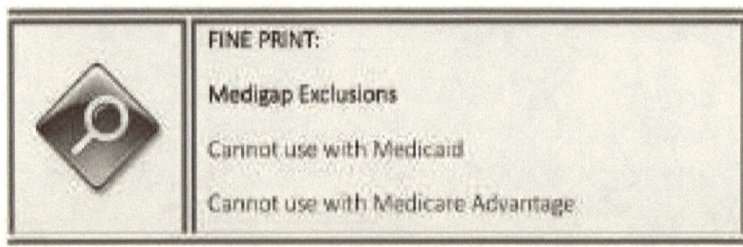

FINE PRINT:

Medigap Exclusions

Cannot use with Medicaid

Cannot use with Medicare Advantage

It is also against the law for a private insurance company to offer you a Medigap plan when you are on Medicare Advantage plan, if do not have plans to change to Original Medicare. They also cannot sell you a new Medigap plan if you already have one and are not planning to cancel your old one. It would be fraudulent to imply that you would need more than one Medigap plan.

You need to look at the PROS and CONS of these plans and decide what will work best for your situation. One good way to get started is to look at your healthcare expenses from the previous year to see where you spent the most money.

Pros and Cons of Medicare Advantage and Medigap Plans

Medicare Advantage	Medigap
PRO: You may gain extra health-care benefits not offered by Original Medicare, such as dental care, vision screening, hearing aids, nursing home coverage, and private nursing care.	CON: You do not gain extra healthcare benefits beyond what Original Medicare offers.
PRO: You may be able to include prescription drug benefits in your plan selection, decreasing how many premiums you have to pay. Note that you would pay Medicare Advantage premiums as well as Part B premiums.	CON: You will have to purchase a Part D plan for prescription drug benefits, adding an additional premium to the Medigap and Original Medicare premiums you would already pay each month.
CON: Medicare Advantage plans still require out-of-pocket expenses, including deductibles, monthly premiums, and co-payments.	PRO: If you have medical conditions that require frequent medical evaluations or hospitalizations, a Medigap plan may save you the most money by covering costly deductibles and co-insurance.
CON: Access to healthcare providers and hospitals is limited by a narrow network.	PRO: You maintain access to all providers and hospitals that accept Original Medicare for payment. The network for Original Medicare is much broader than the ones for Medicare Advantage.

Medicare Savings Programs

There are four Medicare Savings Programs (MSPs) available and they can only be used when you are on Original Medicare. They are run by your state Medicaid office, not by Medicare. If you meet qualifying income and asset levels, an MSP may help you pay deductibles, premiums, co-insurance, and co-payments! That can save a lot of money, all without your needing to pay for a Medigap plan.

Better yet, some states do not even have asset limits! These include Alabama, Arizona, Connecticut, Delaware, District of Columbia, Mississippi, New York, Oregon, and Vermont. They rely on income limits alone. Maine and Minnesota are the only other states that do not follow the Federal guidelines for asset limits but instead set their own limits.

The available Medicare Savings Programs and what they cover are as follows:

Medicare Savings Program	What It Covers
Qualified Disabled and Working Individuals (QDWI)	Part A premiums
Qualifying Individual (QI)	Part B premiums
Qualified Medicare Beneficiary (QMB)	Part A premiums
	Part B premiums, deductibles, co-insurance and co-payments
Specified Low-Income Medicare Beneficiary (SLMB)	Part B premiums

Income includes alimony, annuities, pensions, Railroad Retirement benefits, rental income, Social Security benefits, and Veteran's benefits. It does not include disaster assistance, earned income tax credit payments, home energy assistance, housing assistance, scholarship and educational grants, Supplemental

Nutrition Assistance Program (food stamps), or victim compensation payments.

Medicare Savings Program Eligibility in 2019

	Individual Monthly Income	Individual Assets	Married Monthly Income	Married Assets
QMB	$1,032	$7,560	$1,392	$11,340
SLMB	$1,234	$7,560	$1,666	$11,340
QI	$1,386	$7,560	$1,872	$11,340
QDWI	$4,132	$4,000	$5,572	$6,000

Countable assets include bank accounts (checking, savings, and certificates of deposit), bonds, cars (after your primary vehicle), cash, Individual Retirement Accounts (IRAs), mutual funds, real estate (other than your primary residence), and stocks. They do not include burial plots, burial expenses up to $1,500, furniture and personal items, your primary vehicle, or your primary residence.

Contact your local Medicaid (yes, Medicaid, not Medicare) office for specific requirements in your state.

Extra Help (Part D Low Income Subsidy)

Extra Help, also referred to as the Part D Low Income Subsidy, is similar to a Medicare Savings Program in that it can save you on healthcare costs. The subsidy aims to reduce the cost of prescription drug coverage for those in need, specifically Part D premiums, co-insurance, and co-payments.

There is another benefit to the Extra Help program. If you are one of the unfortunate people who have to pay Part D late penalties, eligibility for Extra Help will wipe them out. This is the only time those penalties can be cancelled.

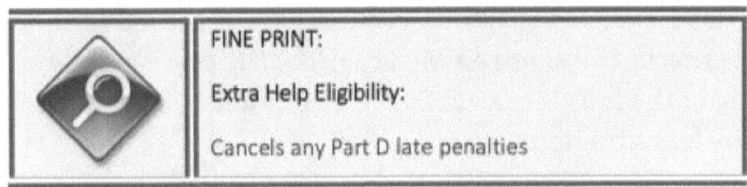

FINE PRINT:

Extra Help Eligibility:

Cancels any Part D late penalties

There are two versions of Extra Help. People who qualify for the full benefit have an income below 135 percent of the federal poverty level (FPL). They will not have to pay a monthly premium for plans that are below the state's standard premium (each state has a different standard). Generic drugs will cost a $3.40 co-pay and brand-name drugs a $8.50 co-pay. After $5,000 is spent out of pocket, no more co-pays will be paid for that year.

The partial benefit (income and asset limits in parentheses in the table above) offers somewhat less but still decreases costs. It applies to people who have an income at or less than 150 percent of FPL. In this case, how much you pay for the monthly premium will depend on your income. You will pay either an $83 deductible or the plan's deductible, whichever is cheaper. For each medication, you will pay a 15 percent co-insurance or the plan's co-pay, whichever is cheaper. After $5,000 is spent out of pocket, you will pay $3.40 for generic drugs, $8.50 for brand-name drugs, or a 5 percent co-insurance, whichever is greater.

	Individual Monthly Income	Individual Assets	Married Monthly Income	Married Assets
Full Extra Help	$1,386	$9,060	$1,872	$14,340
Partial Extra Help	$1,538	$14,100	$2,078	$28,150

Income and assets are counted similar to Medicare Savings Programs, but make sure you reach out to your local Medicaid office for specific requirements in your state. It is possible to get on Extra Help even if you do not meet the standard income and asset criteria. If you are on Medicaid, Social Security Income (SSI) or any of the four Medicaid Savings Programs, you automatically qualify for Extra Help.

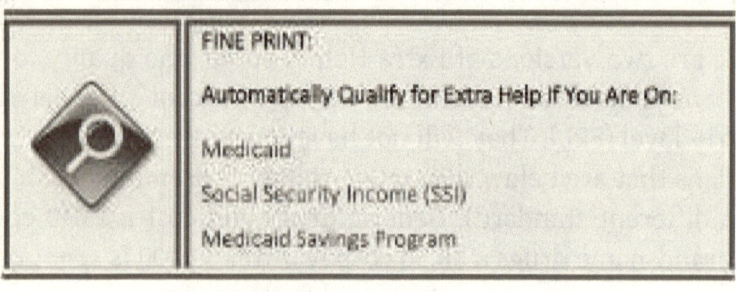

FINE PRINT:

Automatically Qualify for Extra Help If You Are On:

Medicaid

Social Security Income (SSI)

Medicaid Savings Program

Original Medicare vs. Medicare Advantage

Choosing between Original Medicare and Medicare Advantage might seem confusing but don't worry. If you make a choice that doesn't work out for you, you can always change to another plan during the annual Open Enrollment Period (this is distinct from the Medigap Open Enrollment Period which is a one-time event). Medicare's Open Enrollment Period takes place October 15 to December 7 every year.

If you already know that a Medigap plan is right for you, your decision is easy. You should pick Original Medicare.

If you are living on a low income, your decision may be easy too. This is because you may be eligible for Medicare Savings Programs. These programs could save you thousands of dollars per year on your healthcare costs. You may choose to pick Original Medicare.

Deciding Between Original Medicare and Medicare Advantage

	Original Medicare	Medicare Advantage
Coverage	Part A and Part B, must sign up separately for Part D prescription drug coverage	Covers Part A and Part B but may offer additional benefits, may also include Part D coverage
Medicare Savings Plans	Eligible	Not eligible
Medigap Supplement Plans	Eligible	Not eligible
Network	Unlimited	Limited
Out of Pocket Spending	Unlimited	Capped

Top 6 Questions To Ask Yourself When

Choosing a Medicare Plan

If you still feel stumped about whether Original Medicare or Medicare Advantage is right for you, ask yourself these questions.

1. Do you live in an area where there is a doctor shortage?

You will have better access to physicians across all specialties with Original Medicare than Medicare Advantage. Simply put, Original Medicare gives you access to physicians nationwide. If there is a specific doctor you hope to see, odds are an appointment with that provider will be covered.

This is not necessarily the case with Medicare Advantage plans. These plans only cover providers within their designated network and will make you pay more for out of network providers, if they pay at all. Plan networks are limited to a specific region. If you move, you will need to get a new Medicare Advantage plan based on your new location.

The federal government requires that Medicare Advantage plans have enough providers in their network to care for their beneficiaries. Specifically, 90 percent of beneficiaries must be able to access care within set travel time and distance constraints (varied based on rural or urban regions) for at least one provider or facility for a given specialty. That being the case, there is no guarantee that the one provider in question will have appointments available or is even accepting new patients. Worse, what if you are in the 10 percent of beneficiaries outside those time and distance criteria? There could be significant hardships in accessing care when you need it.

The reality is that many networks remain inadequate, especially in areas where there are physician shortages. It is estimated that 1 in 3 Medicare Advantage networks is too narrow, representing less than 30 percent of the physicians in a given county.

You will need to decide whether or not the benefits of a Medicare Advantage plan outweigh possible access issues based on where you live.

2. Are you generally healthy and using minimal healthcare services?

Why would you want to pay more when you can pay less? Original Medicare may be all that you need. Paying an added premium for Medicare Advantage may not give you added benefit.

You will have to decide whether or not it is worth supplementing Original Medicare with a Medigap plan to avoid paying more if you develop conditions in the future.

3. Are there services that Original Medicare does not cover that you need?

Remember that Original Medicare does not cover everything. Specifically, it does not pay for corrective lenses, dentures, or hearing aids. If you need one of these high priced items, Original Medicare is going to leave you in the lurch.

In these cases, a Medicare Advantage plan may be the choice for you. Keep in mind that not every plan will offer coverage for these items so be on the lookout for a plan that covers the specific services you need. Also, remember that coverage for Medicare Advantage plans can change every year. Do not assume your plan will continue to cover the same services from year to year. You may need to switch plans during the Open Enrollment Period to assure you get coverage that meets your needs.

4. How much can you afford to pay out of pocket?

Original Medicare has no limit on out of pocket expenses. If you have chronic medical conditions, you could end up paying a lot. Medicare Advantage plans, however, have a maximum out-of-pocket (MOOP) spending limit, an annual cap on your Medicare expenses.

Once you spend the MOOP amount for your Medicare Advantage plan (your monthly premiums do not count towards the MOOP), the plan is responsible for covering 100% of Medicare-approved costs for the rest of the year. The out-of-pocket maximum varies from plan to plan and may change from year to year. Plans with a low MOOP are likely to have higher premiums and deductibles. You will have to decide which will save you more money in the end.

5. Do you travel a lot?

Lots of people like to travel. Whether you travel within or outside the United may determine whether Original Medicare or Medicare Advantage is right for you.

Domestic travel may steer you towards Original Medicare. Medicare Advantage plans are limited to a local network. Care received even during domestic travel could cost you a lot more simply because it is not in your network. People who live in different parts of the country over the course of the year would be at a disadvantage. Original Medicare, on the other hand, offers you nationwide access to health care.

If you choose Original Medicare, international travel could cost you a pretty penny if you required health care. You could supplement Original Medicare with a Medigap plan to cover expenses for emergency care you receive in a foreign country.

Alternatively, some Medicare Advantage plans have a foreign travel benefit. Coverage may be limited as discussed earlier in this chapter.

6. Do you have chronic medical conditions that require frequent care?

Certain medical conditions are more prone to complications or flare ups. Consider Alzheimer's disease, coronary artery disease, congestive heart failure, chronic obstructive pulmonary disease (COPD), chronic kidney disease, diabetes mellitus, and hypertension, to name a few.

The cost for care can be high. Treatment of heart disease accounts for roughly $1 for every $6 spent on healthcare in the United States. Diabetes cost the country $327 billion in direct medical costs and reduced productivity in 2017. The Alzheimer's Association estimated the direct costs for Alzheimer's disease and other dementias to be $277 billion in 2018, $186 billion of that paid by Medicare and Medicaid. Cancer costs our health system $171 billion a year and we spend $81 billion on arthritis, $56 billion on asthma, and $33 billion on stroke. How much of those costs do you pay?

If you have a medical condition that could require frequent care, you will want to choose a Medicare situation that will save you as much money as possible.

If you have a lot of office visits or hospitalizations, a Medigap plan may save you money by paying off costly deductibles and co-insurance. That means signing up for Original Medicare instead of Medicare Advantage.

However, Medicare Advantage plans could be a good deal because they put a cap on out-of-pocket spending. Please know that these caps do not include what you pay for your monthly premiums. Depending on the specific plan you choose, Medicare Advantage may be a reasonable approach to keep costs down.

How do you decide between the two? It is a math game. How much would you spend on Medigap premiums and how does that dollar amount compare to the Medicare Advantage spending cap? If the Medigap premiums are less than the Medicare Advantage out-of-pocket cap, that may be the overall better deal.

Top 5 Mistakes People Make With Medicare

Advantage

There are no "bad" Medicare Advantage plans out there, but there are plans that may be better for you based on what they offer and how much they cost. Everyone has different needs. Although you will be able to change your plan during the Open Enrollment Period, the hope is that you will pick a "good" plan this year and will not have to wait a whole year to get another one. To find a plan that best meets your needs, avoid the following mistakes.

1. You do not read the Annual Notice of Change for your plan.

At the end of every year, before Medicare Open Enrollment season, your Medicare Advantage plan will send out an Annual Notice of Change. This document outlines what changes are coming in the new year regarding costs and coverage. Too many people do not read the fine print. Premiums, deductibles, and co-payments do not come cheap and price hikes could surprise you come January 1 when the new plan kicks. Losing coverage for services or medications you use on a regular basis would cost you more in out of pocket expenses. Make sure that your existing plan is going to meet your needs in the new year.

2. You do not choose a plan with Part D prescription drug coverage.

People who do not take medications, or who take minimal medications, may chose not to sign up for a Medicare Advantage plan with Part D coverage. Unless you have creditable drug coverage from another source (employer-sponsored health plans, Indian Health Service, Program of All-Inclusive Care for the Elderly, TRICARE, or Veteran's Health benefits), you could be faced with a lifetime of Part D late penalties when you finally do sign up. Creditable coverage means that the drug coverage is as good as Medicare. Your other health plans must notify you if they meet this standard so you can make an informed decision to sign up for Part D.

3. You sign up for the same plan as your spouse or someone you know.

Many people sign up for a specific health plan based on recommendations from people they know. Maybe a friend or neighbor or even your spouse has had a good experience with a plan. Some people may choose a plan based on its brand name and reputation. For many married couples, it is a matter of convenience to use the same insurance company. While these recommendations could steer you to quality plans, your health is unique to you. Your friends and family may not be on the same medications or use the same doctors. You need to find a plan tailored to your individual situation.

4. You do not switch plans to keep your doctors.

Unlike Original Medicare, which covers doctors nationwide, Medicare Advantage plans work in local networks. Networks can change at any time. That means a Medicare plan could drop a provider from its network, not because there are any issues with the provider per se but because there is a disagreement over contractual requirements. If you want to save money and keep the doctors you know and trust, or if there is a doctor you want to go to that is not in your current network, you may want to pick a plan that includes that doctor in its network. Otherwise, you will pay more for your visits, if they are covered at all.

5. You do not shop around for the best deal.

Having the "perfect" plan this year does not mean it will be the perfect plan for you next year. While we hope insurances companies have a goal to provide quality health care, their main intention is to turn a profit. With dollars and cents running the show, insurers are competing with each other in the market and this could work to your advantage. Do not take the path of least resistance and automatically keep your current plan. Take the time to see how other plans compare on costs and pick the one that will give you the best care while saving you the most money.

Professional Reference:

If you have any questions at all, do not hesitate to email or call Roxanne Robertson. She is a verified Medicare insurance consultant, licensed in over 40 states. Roxanne specializes in current Medicare options, and resources which has personally helped thousands of Medicare recipients just like you. In addition her service is free.

She can be reached at:

Roxanne@medigapselect.com

Or directly on her personal cell (913)-592-1291 text is also an option.

9:00 A.M - 6:00 P.M Monday-Saturday